FINDING *Hope* in the STORM

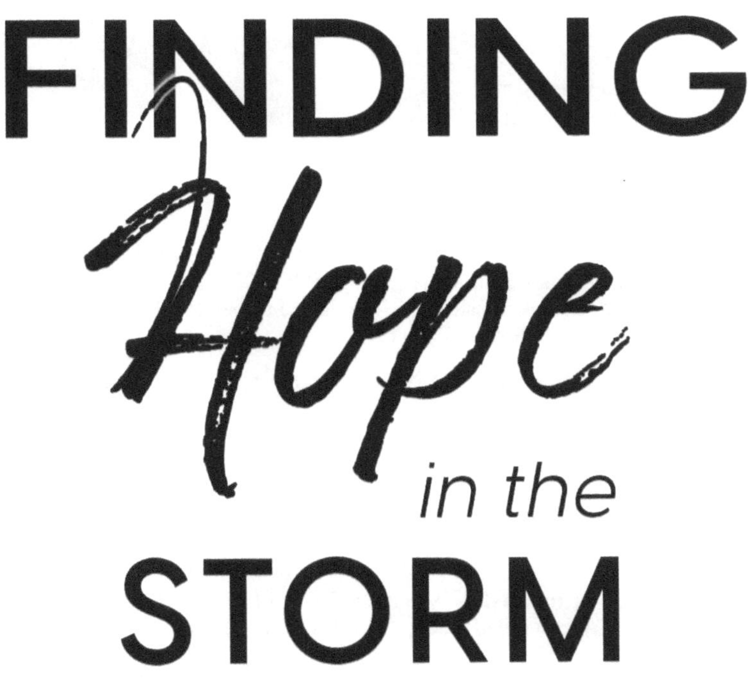

My Journey Through Breast Cancer . . .
Strength-Building Devotions

VICKI EARHART

To anyone experiencing a journey of suffering.
May you find hope and comfort in Jesus.

CONTENTS

ACKNOWLEDGMENTS

My heartfelt thanks go to so many who stood with me throughout this journey. . . .

My husband, David, remained determined that we would make it through this trial. He prayed constantly. He read God's Word to me and sang to me through many sleepless nights. So many times, he encouraged me, "We will have more years to enjoy together." His steadfast understanding and prayers were the biggest help to get me through the discouragement and fears that cancer brought.

My sons and their wives, Shon and Michelle, Chris and Amy, steadfastly prayed and provided words of encouragement, sending daily devotions and Christian music to me. These messages helped me focus on God's strength and power. Both sons were with me when my hair was shaved, providing support and encouragement. They waited with their dad in the parking lot during my first chemo and greeted me with a hug as I came out of the hospital. Their steadfast love was a light of Jesus to me. They encouraged me to fight the battle and continue to live and see my grandchildren grow. Regularly, each of them called to say, "I love you. We are not ready for anything to happen to you!" They prayed for and with me often, asking God for healing and strength. What a blessing to have children who believe in the Lord's power!

And the encouragement from my six grandchildren—Sheldon, Larkin, Ava, Silas, Sawyer, and Cora—meant so much. Each of them (ages three to seventeen) brought me many blessings during my journey.

I can't begin to express how much the support and love from my parents, Charles and Marylyn King; my brother and sister-in-law, Jeff and Angela King; and my nieces have blessed me. They called often and came to visit regularly.

Many prayer warriors have supported me in so many ways—family, friends, and people I've never met. Their prayers carried me to the foot of Jesus many times!

Karen Weigand has been such a blessing to me! As my editor and literary advisor, she was wonderful to work with. Her encouragement reminded me this was my journey . . . but God's story of hope.

I was lifted up daily by an army of prayer warriors who asked God to provide strength and healing. And he protected me and gave me peace in the battle of sickness!

INTRODUCTION

I was a busy, healthy woman in my sixties. I walked three to four miles several times a week and played pickleball regularly—along with lifting weights and bowling. Retired from fifty-two years of nursing, I was heavily involved in church and other activities. I loved spending time with my family and friends.

Then four words changed everything: *It looks like cancer.*

This devotional is about my breast cancer journey. I want to share my story, hoping it will encourage anyone going through cancer or any difficult illness to have *hope.* Hope placed in Jesus. God showed me countless times throughout my journey that he was walking with me. He held my hand throughout the course, comforting me and encouraging me. He provided peace, protection, and strength to get me through the days of tests, treatments, and sickness.

When this journey began, I started journaling every day, and I am sharing those thoughts in this book. It includes most of my journal notes throughout my eighteen months of cancer treatments in 2021 and 2022. The fears, pain, and tears—and the Scriptures that brought me hope. As you read this, may you be comforted by the fact that you are not alone when you experience fear, doubts, sadness, and more. That's normal for someone on this kind of journey, but I do so want you to experience hope as well. Hope in Jesus. Hope in his love for you. Hope in his Word.

Sometimes, especially when we are overwhelmed by fear, pain, and what-ifs, we may not see the signs of his strength or protection. But God's glorious love and blessings are around us daily if we look with an open heart. Jesus has promised us he will never leave us. We can count on him even when we don't feel his presence.

As you read the following pages, I pray you are encouraged. I pray you will see God's signs of holding you up. May he give you strength and peace if you are in the battle of cancer, sickness, or other difficulties of life or if you are a caregiver for someone who is.

Look for the hope he is offering you.

HOW TO USE THIS BOOK

I encourage you to use this book in whatever way works best for you. Each short chapter includes something from my journey, thoughts for reflection, and a varying amount of space for you to write your thoughts.

You may want to read one chapter and meditate on it for a few days before moving ahead. You may want to read straight through and then go back and spend more time on the pages that are most helpful at the moment. Use whatever pace and plan work best for you.

I do hope you will meditate on the Scriptures as they speak to you. At the end of the book, you'll find a Scripture index to remind you of the Bible verses I used and where they can be found in the book.

I encourage you to consider starting your own journal. Journaling helped me in so many ways. It was a way to express my fears and frustrations. It helped draw my focus to Jesus as I found Scriptures that ministered to me. It helped me keep track of side effects and things my doctors told me. And now it has helped me share my experience with you.

May God bless you and strengthen you on your journey— and fill you with hope.

1

IT LOOKS LIKE CANCER

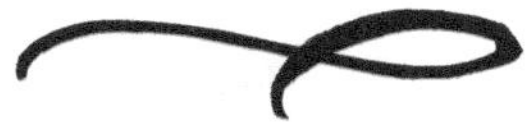

It was Easter Sunday, April 4, 2021. While taking my shower that morning, I noticed a round quarter-size indentation on my right breast. I thought back to the previous December when I had been playing pickleball and one of the balls hit me in the breast. The spot had remained swollen and sore for months—and now, this. My mind shouted, *You must call the doctor as soon as possible!*

Frightening what-ifs invaded my mind, but I determined to set them aside as my husband, David, and I enjoyed a wonderful day celebrating Jesus's resurrection at worship services and lunch at our home with our family. When everyone had left, I finally told David what I had discovered.

The next morning when I called my doctor's office for an appointment, they said to come right in. My primary care doctor saw me first—and then the flurry began. She sent me directly to the hospital for a mammogram and ultrasound.

Then David and I waited—eager for results but dreading them at the same time. The radiologist walked into the room. "I don't see anything abnormal in your left breast. All lymph nodes look fine. There is a lump in the right breast—and it looks like cancer."

My head began to reel. *What am I hearing? What am I to do?* I was confused. Afraid. I had been a nurse for fifty-two years, and my thoughts quickly turned to the next steps. *I don't know who I want for surgery. Do I get treatment here in Joplin? Do I go to Kansas University or MD Anderson Cancer Center in Houston? What should I do?*

As David and I left the radiologist's office, they gave me an appointment for a breast biopsy in a week. *A week. How can I wait that long?* Fear tightened its grip. My world was turning upside down with confusion. I knew Satan was very much alive, and he was after my mind, my heart, and my soul.

> Stay alert! Watch out for your great enemy, the devil. He prowls around like a roaring lion, looking for someone to devour. Stand firm against him, and be strong in your faith.
>
> — 1 Peter 5:8–9

I knew standing firm in the faith meant focusing on Jesus and his Word. Scriptures began running through my mind—Scriptures of hope like this one:

> Give your burdens to the Lord, and he will take care of you. He will not permit the godly to slip and fall.

> — PSALM 55:22

Reflections

Our life had suddenly taken a heart-stopping turn. Overnight everything focused on the diagnosis. On the what-ifs. On the what-to-do's.

Can you identify? Have you received a cancer diagnosis? Or equally devastating news?

Like me, you may be reeling with fear and confusion. Please don't let those haunting emotions overwhelm you. I would like to share my journey with you. To tell you how I found hope. The first step is to focus on Jesus. He knows you. He loves you. And he cares.

And so, Lord, where do I put my hope? My only hope is in you.

> — PSALM 39:7

Lord, I don't understand what is happening. I don't know what to do, but you do. Please help me trust you—your way, your plan, your love.

2

A CROSS IN A TREE

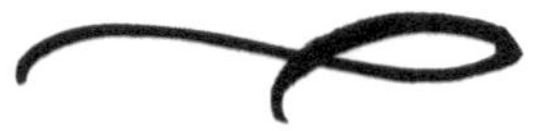

Still reeling with fear, I had so many questions. I called two women I knew who had experienced cancer. One had gone to MD Anderson in Houston and the other to Kansas University (KU). I needed to hear from someone who had been there, so I asked both about the care they had received. And, of course, I asked them to pray.

The next day, April 6, my primary care doctor called to express her sadness and concern and encourage me to find the top care I could. She promised to be praying for me. Then calls and text messages from friends began to pour in—all expressing love and concern and committing to pray. That meant so much.

I slept some that night but then awoke with my mind spinning and my heart pounding. *Will I have a mastectomy?*

Maybe I won't need chemo or radiation since we caught it so early. Right? Or had we? How can we afford this? Will I die?

The fear was turning into panic. I knew I had to somehow find hope.

My thoughts turned to a morning weeks before. I had been sitting at the kitchen table eating oatmeal and looking out the window at the heavily wooded area behind our yard. Suddenly one of the trees caught my eye. There seemed to be a round circle with a cross in the tree trunk. I quickly took a picture with my phone and enlarged it. Yes, it was a cross! When David came into the kitchen, he could see it too, even though we were seventy-five feet away. It looked as if someone had carved out the bark and cut a cross in the tree. But when we walked to the tree to examine it, we realized no one had carved the cross—the tree had grown that way!

I began to wonder if God had been preparing me for what he knew I'd be facing in just a few weeks. Did he want to remind me of his love—or maybe of Jesus's suffering? To remind me that God was with Jesus and gave him strength through his anguish on the cross? I believe he was reassuring me he would give me strength for whatever was to come.

I knew the only way I could find hope in the days ahead was in God. In his Word.

Wow! I realized that through that cross in the tree, God had reminded me that Jesus loved me so much he died for me. He wanted me to remember how he had carried Jesus through the terrible pain of crucifixion and afterward raised him from the dead for eternal life. Because of that, we too can have eternal life. I knew that whatever lay ahead, he would be with me. He would strengthen me. And he would bring good.

Throughout the ordeal that was to come, I still had fear … I sometimes didn't know how I could go on … but then I would remember God was with me. And because of that, I could live with hope.

Reflections

You may be facing a journey that will include times of sickness, pain, fear, and confusion. I hope you will find that even through the most difficult times, you can find hope by trusting in Jesus. By looking to God's Word for strength and peace.

God loves you. He may show you his love through friends or family who care. He may show it through His Word. He may show you that through a cross in a tree! Or he may show you that in a unique way he has planned just for you. Keep your eyes on him.

Lord, I wait for you; you will answer, Lord my God.

— Psalm 38:15 NIV

My Thoughts

3

EVEN IF . . .
WE WILL TRUST HIM

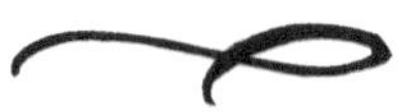

April 8, 2021. David and I FaceTimed our sons and their wives to give them the news. We were so touched by the love and concern expressed through their tears, encouragement, and prayers. Our older son, Shon, shared examples of God as the great healer and miracle worker, reminding us of Bible examples. He said he was thankful my faith was strong enough to use this for God's glory.

We agreed to pray for no cancer. But if it was cancer, we would trust and know God is the great healer! We would trust him for direction and strength. Our sons and David each prayed. The daughters-in-law and I cried.

April 9. Our younger son, Chris, called to thank us for letting him know what was going on. His loving call was followed by one from Shon. He wanted to know how I was doing.

I had a meltdown—one of joy and gratitude. As our sons were growing up, we had taught them from God's Word and tried to live the Word as much as we could before them. Now they were both adults, teaching their children about God's ways. And here they were walking beside me in faith, encouraging me during this difficult time. *Oh, Lord, thank you so much.*

> I have no greater joy than to hear that my children are walking in the truth.

> — 3 John 1:4 NIV

I began to realize how important their faith was to me as I began this journey with so many unknowns. I knew they would hold me before God, continually asking him to bring me peace, strength, and healing. I believed they would accept God's plan, whatever it was.

Both our daughters-in-law were a Godsend as well. Amy, a nurse, had already begun researching what doctor at MD Anderson I should request. She said I should get a CT or PET scan. A CT scan would check for masses in other parts of my body. A PET scan is more helpful for detecting lymph node involvement and metastasis.

However, we knew they may not do the PET scan until they had the biopsy results—another wait!

Our other daughter-in-law, Michelle, sent me an encouraging note. "You are strong, special, awesome, tough, loved—and not alone! You are supported, worth it, amazing! You are brave and courageous. You are a fighter!"

With my family's support, I must find hope.

Reflections

My family reminded me that even if it was cancer, we must trust God for his plan. If you have been diagnosed with cancer (or any other serious illness), please remember God has not abandoned you. He is right there with you. And as you keep your eyes on him, I believe he will send you encouraging reminders of his love, as he did for me. Encouragement may come from your family . . . from friends . . . from someone at church . . . or even from a stranger.

Of course, the best place to find truth and hope is in the Bible. Find Scriptures that speak to you. Read them every day—maybe several times a day. Write them on Post-its or index cards and tape them around your house or office. Speak them often. These are some that helped me. . . . I hope they will speak to you as well.

He gives strength to the weary and increases the power of the weak.

— Isaiah 40:29 NIV

The Lord delights in those who fear him, who put their hope in his unfailing love.

— Psalm 147:11 NIV

— *My Thoughts* —

4

FROM THE KNOWN TO THE UNKNOWN

April 9, 2021. *Lord, I know you have blessed me with the hope of heaven. I know I will be with you for all eternity, but I am not ready to leave this life on earth. Is that how Jesus felt when he asked you to let his cup pass from him? Did he want to stay to do more ministry? Did he not want to go through the pain? And yet, he chose your will, not his. What is going to happen to me? How long? How much pain?*

I was beginning to struggle with fear. I still believed in God, but I wanted direction. A plan. My life was moving in a completely new direction. I needed to get busy canceling all the old plans—bowling, pickleball, Bible studies, committees, board meetings. I was leaving the known to enter a great big unknown. I needed to find hope.

And then a note arrived from a friend reminding me of a song about hope. A text from Amy assured me of her prayers and love. And then a gift on my porch—a small frame with a Scripture about hope.

> Rejoice in hope, be patient in tribulation, be constant in prayer.
>
> — ROMANS 12:12 ESV

Yes, Lord. Thank you for these reminders that with you, there is always hope.

Encouraging text messages of prayers continued streaming in. *I must have hope!*

April 11. Another message of hope from a friend. *I must have hope!* Yet another message: "It's not wasted, friend, this trial, this suffering, this fire you're going through. The Lord promises purpose in all of it, for the purifying of your faith and the praise of his name when you see his faithfulness through it." Oh, such wonderful words of hope!

I began to wonder about *hope*. What is it? Is it trusting in things you can't understand? I went to a dictionary: Hope is "to cherish a desire with anticipation."[1] It involves trusting. Hope is imagining that there is something to believe and trust in. The same dictionary told me that trust is confidence and dependence on something or someone and having hope in it or them.[2] Trust is a feeling. It is an incredibly powerful emotion and a natural part of human relationships. We must do the work to have hope!

At this point, my cherished desire was to have the strength to walk through whatever lay ahead. To be healed. And I had no doubt about the object of my trust: Jesus. I believed and trusted in him. I had confidence in him and knew I needed to depend on him.

Reflections

Where are you in your journey? Like me, you may be experiencing fear of the unknown. Fear of the pain. Fear of leaving this earth and your loved ones.

Ask God to help you let go of the things you cannot change. Ask him to make your experience a beautiful gift of hope for others. Keep your eyes on Jesus, asking him to give you the strength to run the race set before you.

I will look fear in the face. I will live through this horror! I must do the things I think I cannot do! God's power is going before me!

I can do all things [which He has called me to do] through Him who strengthens and empowers me [to fulfill His purpose—I am self-sufficient in Christ's sufficiency; I am ready for anything and equal to anything through Him who infuses me with inner strength and confident peace].

— Philippians 4:13 AMP

What is your cherished desire? What do you hope for with anticipation? And who are you trusting to fulfill that desire? Where is your hope?

I found so much comfort from Psalm 121. I hope you will too. I encourage you to read it and meditate on it.

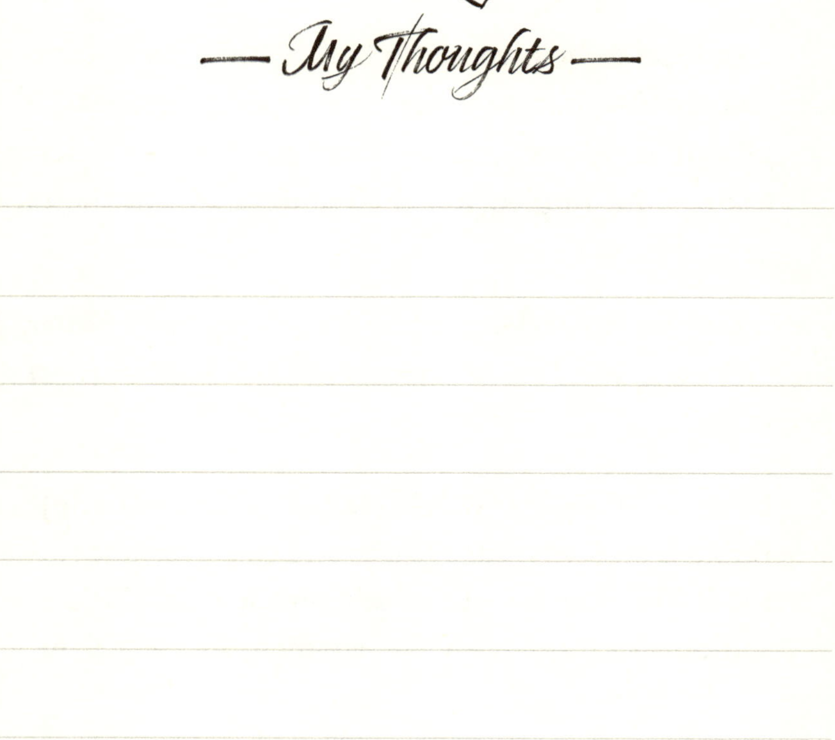

5

FAITH THROUGH DISAPPOINTMENT

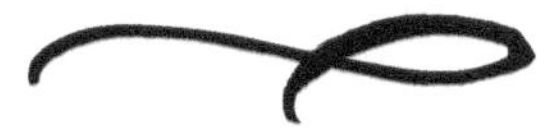

Amy's OB/GYN made a recommendation for my MD Anderson surgeon. I began filling out papers online for an appointment at the MD Anderson Cancer Center in Houston, Texas. They answered within a few minutes, assuring me they would contact me within twenty-four hours with appointment information. I sent them all my medical records electronically. Living in this day of fast communication was a praise!

April 12, 2021. The day had arrived for my biopsy at Mercy Hospital in Joplin. I received many text messages of prayers that morning. *How could I not have hope? But what do I hope? Hope for no cancer? Hope they find what is wrong? Hope . . . what?*

After several numbing shots, the doctor removed some tissue and put markers in those places to indicate where the tissue had been taken. The procedure took about an hour and a half. My heart was sad when he said with confidence, "I am sure this is cancer."

I was filled with despair. *Now I have no hope it's not cancer. But I can hope that they can treat it and get it all out in surgery. I can hope the cancer is only in that one breast and nowhere else.*

Leaving the hospital, I texted some prayer warriors: "I just got done. It was a long procedure, but I remained calm. Thank you for praying to get me through this far! The doctor believes it is cancer." Many responded with encouragement.

I thought of God's promises to be with me. This verse was a strong reminder:

> "Don't be afraid, for I am with you. Don't be discouraged, for I am your God. I will strengthen you and help you. I will hold you up with my victorious right hand."
>
> — Isaiah 41:10

Reflections

Wherever you are in your journey, you may be facing disappointments along the way. It is so easy to let fear take over. I found I had to be proactive in overcoming fear. I believe God filled those around me with encouraging words. I also had to deliberately focus on Jesus and his promises. Although it was far from easy, I had to choose faith over fear. I encourage you to choose faith today, and every day.

Faith that nothing can separate you from God's love.

No, despite all these things, overwhelming victory is ours through Christ, who loved us. And I am convinced that nothing can ever separate us from God's love. Neither death nor life, neither angels nor demons, neither our fears for today nor our worries about tomorrow—not even the powers of hell can separate us from God's love. No power in the sky above or in the earth below—indeed, nothing in all creation will ever be able to separate us from the love of God that is revealed in Christ Jesus our Lord.

— ROMANS 8:37–39

Faith that no matter what happens, God is with you.

"When you go through deep waters, I will be with you. When you go through rivers of difficulty, you will not drown. When you walk through the fire of oppression, you will not be burned up; the flames will not consume you."

— ISAIAH 43:2

Faith in God's strength—not your own.

God is our refuge and strength, always ready to help in times of trouble. So we will not fear when earthquakes come and the mountains crumble into the sea. Let the oceans roar and foam. Let the mountains tremble as the waters surge!

— Psalm 46:1–3

HE HELD MY HAND

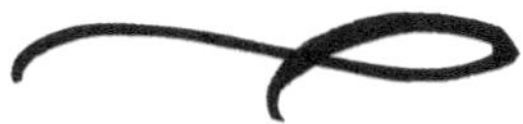

April 14, 2021. David and I went for my biopsy follow-up. This time it was no surprise to hear the doctor confirm that it was cancer. He went on to say, "We don't know what type till we get the lab report next Monday. You will get that report at your visit with your surgeon."

Then the sweet nurse navigator took over for an hour to explain my cancer. It was about an inch, which she said was big. She explained all the programs for financial needs and gave me several cancer books, a tote bag, and a notebook. She told us about the possible options I would have when the final report came. Then she prayed for us. What a blessing to receive prayer from those taking care of me!

The nurse gave me my next appointment with a surgeon and had Mercy fax my records to MD Anderson. She also gave me hard copies and CDs of my records. What a help it was getting all that done at this point! I knew that should help me get an appointment at MD.

As I left the hospital I began crying. *I am so afraid! I am confused about how this happened! Why me, Lord? Why? Why?*

As we left the parking lot, I texted my boys about the results. Then I called my brother, Jeff, and we headed to Mom and Dad's to tell them. Mom cried and Dad looked so sad, but both talked and asked questions. After getting her composure, Mom stood up and said, "Let's pray." Mom and Dad both prayed; then David and I did. Thank God for godly parents! This was all super, super hard, but they encouraged me to have hope.

As we left my parents' home, my tears began to flow again. I knew God was the great healer and giver of life—but I was so afraid. Afraid of the pain. Afraid of the what-ifs. My mind dreamed up problems that may never happen. Over and over, I said, "God is my Lord. He will walk with me through this. I must have hope."

Encouragement continued to flow in from prayer warriors. I already mentioned how Isaiah 41:10 ministered to me. Throughout the journey ahead, this verse was sent to me many times. Throughout the months of tests and treatments, I said it over and over. I had a vision—I could see God stretching his big right hand down and holding mine. He held my hand through every test, biopsy, and treatment. Later I repeated this verse as I had radiation treatments. I said it over and over as I lay sick on the sofa and on the floor, too ill to make it back to the bed. *I must not fear! I must stay positive in trusting God for healing!*

Reflections

I hope God will minister to you through this verse too. Say it repeatedly. Write it down. Memorize it! Picture him holding your hand.

"Don't be afraid, for I am with you. Don't be discouraged, for I am your God. I will strengthen you and help you. I will hold you up with my victorious right hand."

— Isaiah 41:10

I encourage you to talk to Jesus continually. Focus on him and his love. Ask him for peace in the middle of the storm.

You will keep in perfect peace all who trust in you, all whose thoughts are fixed on you!

— Isaiah 26:3

Say this with me: *Hope is a golden cord connecting me to heaven. This cord helps hold my head up, even when the trials are around me. I trust in Jesus. He is my hope, and his love is all around me. His peace is in his presence as he breathes his peace on me. I have joy because of his unfailing love. Jesus is my hope.*

— My Thoughts —

PRESS ON . . . WITH PEACE

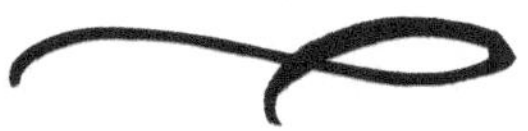

April 15–18, 2021. *Now what do I do as I wait for the next appointment?* I began taking care of responsibilities I had with Bible studies and events. It was overwhelming to make changes in life plans, life routines. I couldn't even tell people when I would be able to start serving again because I had no idea when we would return home from Texas.

I decided to begin by focusing on clothes I would need for hospital stays and surgery. I gathered tops that could be worn after a mastectomy and bought a lounging bed pillow to provide support for my arms and back. I made sure I had robes and house shoes for the hospital stay. I decided I would need clothes for at least six weeks—but I actually had no idea what would be done and when.

I spent time with friends each day. I changed my schedules and gave others my responsibilities in Bible studies, organizations, bowling, and church. I made plans for our home care while we'd be gone. David and I did some spring cleaning and scheduled lawn and landscaping services for the summer.

So many things to think about. We had two weeks to prepare for six weeks away from home.

Loving, encouraging, prayerful texts and calls continued to cover me with the love and support of friends and family.

The sermon at our church that Sunday (Christ's Church of Oronogo) was on *peace*—our joy enables us to stand firm in the Lord.

> Always be full of joy in the Lord. I say it again—rejoice! Let everyone see that you are considerate in all you do. Remember, the Lord is coming soon. Don't worry about anything; instead, pray about everything. Tell God what you need, and thank him for all he has done. Then you will experience God's peace, which exceeds anything we can understand. His peace will guard your hearts and minds as you live in Christ Jesus.
>
> — Philippians 4:4–7

I was reminded to press on. I knew I was to have peace about my life journey and to guard my heart every day.

Reflections

I am God's child, and I will not allow Satan to steal my joy. I will use God's strength and fix my eyes on Jesus. I am hoping in the Lord. He is the giver of my days!

You may be experiencing fear. That's only natural when you are facing cancer and all the what-ifs it brings. But it is so important you don't give in to the fears. Don't quit! Don't give up! Speak God's Word to overcome. He will help you. Speak his name and call on him. Refuse to allow Satan to steal your joy and your faith! Tell him this: "Get behind me, Satan, for I am going to be victorious! I will hold my banner high. God is fighting inside me, and he will give me victory!"

So humble yourselves before God. Resist the devil, and he will flee from you. Come close to God, and God will come close to you.

— JAMES 4:7–8

Stay alert! Watch out for your great enemy, the devil. He prowls around like a roaring lion, looking for someone to devour. Stand firm against him, and be strong in your faith.

— 1 PETER 5:8–9

Lord, bring me peace each day to replace the fears of what could be.

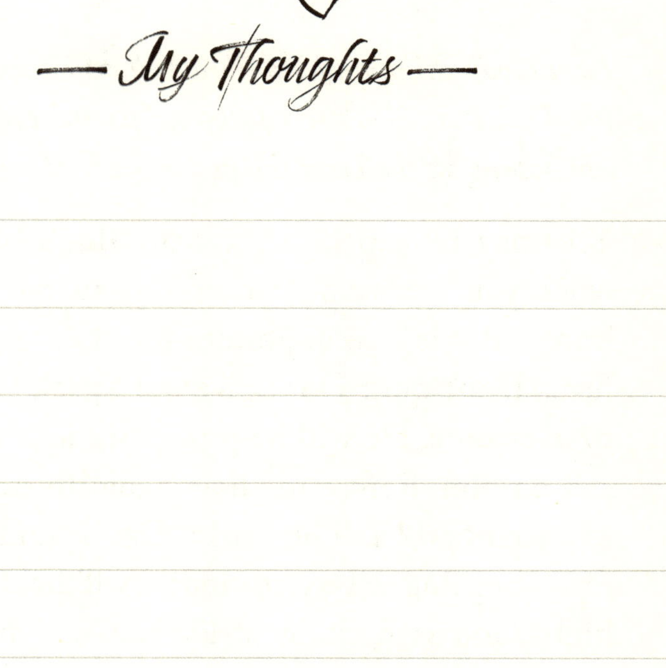

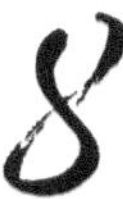

PRAY FOR ONE ANOTHER

Many friends at church prayed with me that Sunday. They hugged me, and we shed tears together. Throughout my cancer journey, it was such a blessing to have their support and prayer to help carry me along. We walked together in faith. I depended on their prayers the most when I was the weakest.

Lord, do you hear these friends' prayers? I am so thankful for them. Please keep a hedge of protection around me! Hold me up! I am needing my family and friends! I am with sorrow, and I want them to be close and pray with me.

God wants us to pray for one another.

> Confess your sins to each other and pray for each other so that you may be healed. The earnest prayer

of a righteous person has great power and produces wonderful results.

— JAMES 5:16

Share each other's burdens, and in this way obey the law of Christ.

— GALATIANS 6:2

Pray in the Spirit at all times and on every occasion. Stay alert and be persistent in your prayers for all believers everywhere.

— EPHESIANS 6:18

I urge you, first of all, to pray for all people. Ask God to help them; intercede on their behalf, and give thanks for them.

— 1 TIMOTHY 2:1

We got together with our small home care group that day for lunch. They all prayed over me. In the evening we had dinner with friends. They prayed for me, asking God to heal me. These prayer warriors brought me hope for God's healing. Hope he would walk daily with me as I went through the tests and treatments. Hope I would one day return home from the treatments in Texas.

I was so blessed to have Christian friends walking beside me.

Reflections

God helped me more than I can ever express through the prayers of friends and family. You too must depend on a team of prayer warriors. If you do not have a group to help lift you up, I urge you to contact a church or cancer support group and ask for prayers. Only God can bring peace and strength to get you through this very hard time of sickness.

At times throughout my journey, God gave me peace. Then fear took over and stole that peace. Each time that happened, I knew I must reach back to God!

No matter how small or big your cancer is, your mind and heart may become depressed. Sadness and fear can cause you to lose hope. Each one of us must get help through the journey! If you don't already have prayer support, please reach out today.

Look to the cross as you go through your journey. Jesus understands physical pain. He understands sorrow.

Walk with a friend who is going through cancer. Seek a friend for yourself if you are going through cancer. Let a friend bring you food, take you to treatment, or come visit. Don't shut out those God is providing to walk with you. Be honest with your family and friends about your fear and pain.

— My Thoughts —

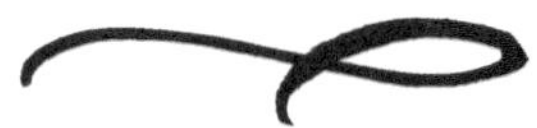

9

OPEN YOUR HEART
TO OTHERS

I messaged my prayer warriors: "It is cancer but not sure what kind. I have an appointment Monday at 3:00 to learn that information. Keep praying for me!"

And the messages of encouragement, prayer, love, and hope continued to flow in.

April 19, 2021. I tried to get a little exercise at the Y. Even there, people came up to me to express their concern and ask how I was doing. One woman, a pharmacist, offered to help me understand my treatment medicines. She also promised to pray for me daily.

That afternoon I met with a surgeon in my hometown. He was positive I would need a bone scan, PET scan, body scan, and labs. Then at least three months of chemo, followed by either a lumpectomy or surgery to remove the breast. If I had a lumpectomy, I would need to have chemo for another year, plus anti-estrogen drugs.

I said I wanted a mastectomy. I also explained I wanted to go to MD Anderson in Houston. He responded that I didn't need to do that but that he would support my getting a second opinion. When I told him my children lived in Houston, he said, "Oh good. That's what you need—to be with family!" From then on, he was very supportive and encouraging.

While I was still in the doctor's office, I received a message from MD Anderson with my appointment details.

Leaving the doctor's office, I sent this message to my prayer warriors:

> Today we talked with a local general surgeon at Mercy Hospital. He said he wanted to do body and bone scans to see if it's into other organs, then begin chemotherapy for three months. After that we would do surgery to remove both breasts and follow up for five years with anti-estrogen meds. I want a second opinion, so we will go to MD Anderson in Houston, Texas, the week of May 3. I have an appointment to see a surgeon there on May 10. I will not have any more tests till we get down there. Every day they will do tests—some I have already had done, but they will do more. Keep praying for God to show his miracle of healing. Also, that it has not spread to any other

organ or anywhere else in my body. Pray it is not in my lymph nodes. Hold me up to the Lord, and ask him to provide direction and clear understanding. I need my prayer warriors, along with my faith, to carry me through this! Love you all.

Once again, the encouraging text messages and prayers helped me so much. They were very touching. Tears began flowing down my face.

That evening we FaceTimed with our kids and talked to my brother, Jeff, providing them with the day's information. I told them about the biopsies and scans I would have in Texas. They would put in an IV infusion port for chemo to begin quickly. I told them how scared I was—worried the cancer would be found elsewhere in my body. Most important, I asked them to pray.

Reflections

I learned that if we open our hearts to those around us, we will find many of them want to help. As you do that, people may not know what to say about your pain and sickness, but many of them will know how to pray.

Please don't hold things in. Be open and honest— especially with those who are praying for you. That will help them know how to pray more specifically. God calls us to pray for and encourage one another.

So we, who are many, are [nevertheless just] one body in Christ, and individually [we are] parts one of another [mutually dependent on each other].

— Romans 12:5 AMP

Carry one another's burdens and in this way you will fulfill the requirements of the law of Christ [that is, the law of Christian love].

— Galatians 6:2 AMP

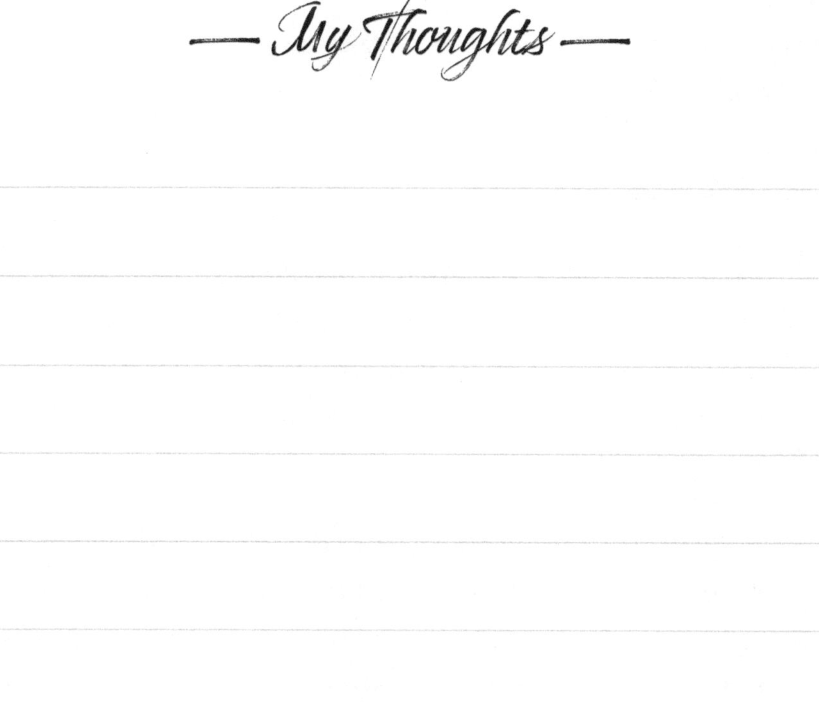

10

IN ALL THINGS GIVE THANKS

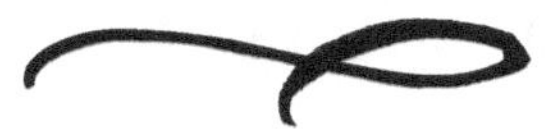

April 21, 2021. *Lord, please fight this battle of cancer! Remove it. Hear the prayers of relatives and friends asking you to fight this sickness and give me life. Lord, today remove any other cancer cells that may be in my body. Keep my cancer local in only one breast. May it seal off and not grow anymore. Lord, may our prayers for healing be heard. I don't like being sick, and I don't like to be whining. I want to live! Live to see my grandchildren at their graduation. Lord, I long to live more years with David as my helpmate and friend. Lord, bless him and give him strength.*

The hospital had given me a book about cancer when I was diagnosed. On this day, I read a page listing things to be thankful for in my circumstances. I found the list interesting—it suggested keeping my mind on the simple things in life that surround me. The alarm clock to awaken me. The cold floors as I get out of bed. Dirty dishes. Laundry. Friends who come to visit. All the good things that help my heart and mind to refocus and keep my mind off how bad things could be. Remember, all these things are a part of living! I gave thanks that I was alive. I gave thanks for all these everyday things around me.

How hard being thankful can be sometimes, but I was alive! *I don't like or want pain, nausea, or separation from family. However, in the days ahead I have my God to give me strength. I must be thankful I can hear others talk, eat food, and enjoy family and all the things around me. My yard and beautiful trees, air to breathe, the sky that brings me peace as I see the clouds forming.*

That evening the elders at our church anointed me with oil and prayed over me.

> Is anyone among you sick? Let them call the elders of the church to pray over them and anoint them with oil in the name of the Lord.
>
> — JAMES 5:14 NIV

Prayers and messages continued.

April 23. I had lunch with a long-time friend, a fellow nurse. We discussed the pros and cons of treatments and drugs. I saw other friends at the restaurant who later texted me to say they would take food to my parents while I was in Texas.

This was another way God was sending me blessings, encouragement, and strength from friends. We must continually look around us and see how God is blessing us, how he speaks peace and strength into our hearts and souls. We must listen to his small whispers.

So many blessings. So much to be thankful for, even in the middle of this storm.

Reflections

We all have lots to be thankful for, no matter what challenges or troubles we may be facing. If we focus on the bad, we will lose sight of the good. God calls us to focus on the positive.

Fix your thoughts on what is true, and honorable, and right, and pure, and lovely, and admirable. Think about things that are excellent and worthy of praise.

— Philippians 4:8

We need to walk in thanksgiving.

In every situation [no matter what the circumstances] be thankful and continually give thanks to God; for this is the will of God for you in Christ Jesus.

— 1 Thessalonians 5:18 AMP

What are you thankful for today? I hope you'll write a list and add to it daily.

54

♡

— *My Thoughts* —

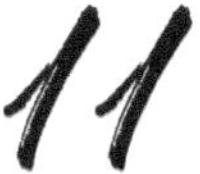

GOD IS WITH YOU

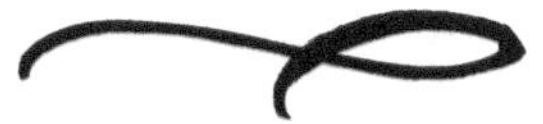

April 24, 2021. I had several cries throughout the day but kept busy wrapping Mother's Day and May birthday gifts so I could give them before leaving for Texas. We would be gone the entire month of May.

That evening we went to dinner with my mom and dad. We picked a nice restaurant where we could relax and talk. I loved being with them. I enjoyed living close to them and being able to have their love in my life, even though I was seventy!

I love my mom so much. She is filled with God's Spirit and prays often. At dinner she gave me a handwritten note.

Don't you know that day dawns after night, showers displace drought, and spring and summer follow winter? Then, have hope! Hope forever for God will not fail you!

— Charles Spurgeon April 25[3]

At church many came and prayed for me or hugged me with words of encouragement. After lunch we came home and began cleaning out flowerbeds and the pantry. I decided to sell my cake decorating pans since I wouldn't be doing any more cake decorating. The mastectomy would prevent me from using my arm for a long time. A friend offered to sell the pans at her flea market. I had several meltdowns as I cleaned them and began crying while packing our suitcases for the trip to Texas.

This was so hard! My heart was hurting and fearful. I didn't want to go through this journey, but I knew we cannot change what God decides. We can plead with him, but he has a plan. We don't control his decisions and power—no matter how good we are or how much we hurt. But he promises to walk with us through the journey. I needed to remember above all else that no matter how bleak things may look, his plans and his timing are always perfect.

More tears. *I am so afraid. Lord, I don't want to die, but I feel as if my life is coming to an end. I pray I can live to see my grandkids grow into adulthood.* I called out to the Lord for strength.

April 25. That night I went to Bible Study Fellowship. The women in my class all laid hands on me and prayed over me. We studied Genesis 47 about blessings through trials. God's Word makes it clear there are many blessings in both good and bad things that happen to us. Throughout the years, I have spent much time in God's Word. Maybe I will never understand some things in my life, but I am so thankful that the Bible has revealed God's great love for me. As I entered this journey, I began applying many Bible stories to my cancer journey. These stories and Scriptures would prove to help me throughout all the struggles ahead. Noah's ark (later you will learn about God reassuring me of his presence through rainbows). The lame man whose friends lowered him though a house rooftop to Jesus for healing. Peter walking on the water to Jesus. Jesus in the garden asking God to take the cup from him. Jesus on the cross.

Reflections

Everyone experiences some form of suffering and pain. Think of the torture Jesus suffered. He was beaten beyond recognition and then suffered the agonies of the cross. Never will anyone suffer as much as he did as he carried the sins of all humankind—out of obedience to the Father and unimaginable unconditional love for us. He suffered not only excruciating physical pain but also the pain of rejection from all those around him.

As you travel this journey, always remember that God is with you. This kind of suffering is beyond our understanding, but we need to trust him—for the journey and for the outcome.

"Do not be afraid or discouraged, for the Lord will personally go ahead of you. He will be with you; he will neither fail you nor abandon you."

— Deuteronomy 31:8

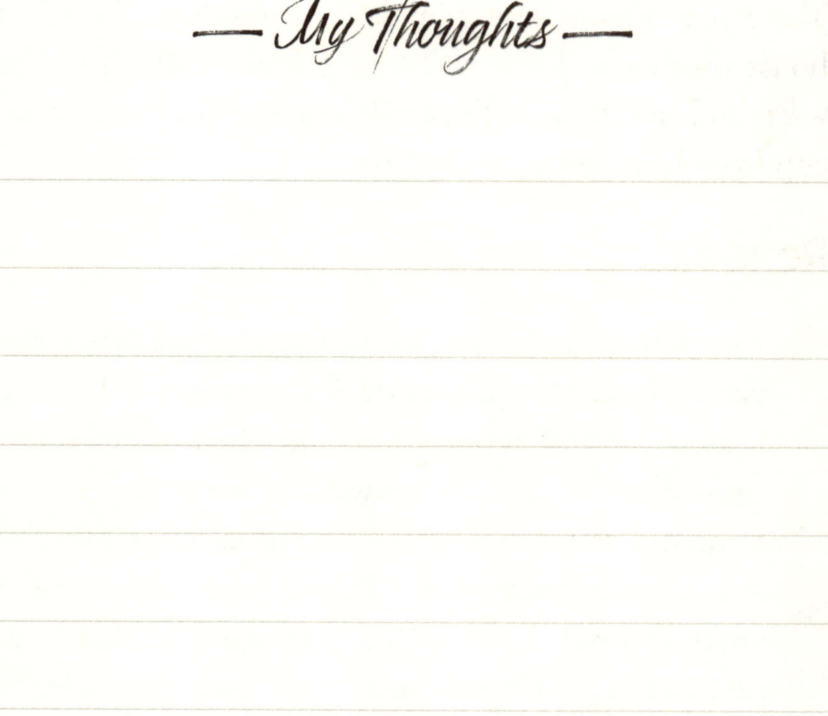

My Thoughts

12

IT IS NOT FOREVER

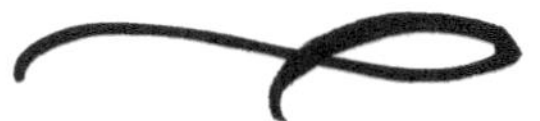

April 27, 2021. Another busy day! David and I were at a board meeting for a local ordination organization when the nurse navigator, Nicole, called from MD Anderson to explain more details about my cancer. She began by describing the anatomy of the breast, where my cancer was in the breast, and how it was spreading. She said it didn't look as if it was in the lymph nodes. They were rechecking some of the tests, especially the HER2 factor. She answered my questions and went on to explain the surgery would be in the downtown main hospital. We could stay at the hotel in the hospital, which has a walkway connecting them. She would make those arrangements when we had a surgery date.

Later that day a friend and I went to look at wigs, and I tried some on. The cost was twelve hundred dollars, but with a prescription from my doctor, our insurance would pay part of that.

I fought back tears. I could not even think about not having any hair, and I was overwhelmed by the cost. *How will I go places with no hair? How long before it will grow back? I sure can't decide about this today!* My friend was a light to keep me positive.

While I was wig shopping, David went to Chick-fil-A and visited with the owner, one of my prayer warriors. She gave him several gift cards for Chick-fil-A meals to use while we were in Texas.

More encouragement came from friends that evening. One had had a lump removed a few months before and had been treated with radiation. Her knowledge and experience were helpful. Another told me she'd received treatment at MD a few years before, and it was the best place in the world!

April 28. I enjoyed time at the Y and played pickleball. David had breakfast with a friend who offered to mentor and support him throughout my cancer journey. One more blessing from God. Another man spending time with him and praying with him would be such an encouragement. He was so positive and encouraging to me, but I was sure he was also afraid and worried about what would happen.

I was in a bowling league and played with my team. We won all three games! What a happy last day for me! We would be gone for the final weeks of the season, and I knew they would be praying for me.

More prayers. More encouraging messages. A message from daughter-in-law Michelle was especially uplifting.

Reflections

One friend sent a Scripture I've mentioned before. This passage helped me a lot in the months ahead. I know it will help you too.

You will keep in perfect peace all who trust in you, all whose thoughts are fixed on you! Trust in the Lord always, for the Lord God is the eternal Rock.

— Isaiah 26:3–4

I also received a special message from my mom. She shared these words inspired by God: "I am doing things you can't understand. Trust Me. I am taking care of you. Watch to see what I will do." She also reminded me of the words of Jesus in this Scripture:

"So you have sorrow now, but I will see you again; then you will rejoice, and no one can rob you of that joy."

— John 16:22

I was so afraid. And I would suffer greatly throughout the treatments. It was far from easy, but God saw me through. He will see you through your journey too. You are passing through—it will not forever. And God won't leave you for even a second. Even those times you don't feel his presence, he is with you. You can know that because he has promised.

"So be strong and courageous! Do not be afraid and do not panic before them. For the Lord your God will personally go ahead of you. He will neither fail you nor abandon you."

— Deuteronomy 31:6

13

HE CARES

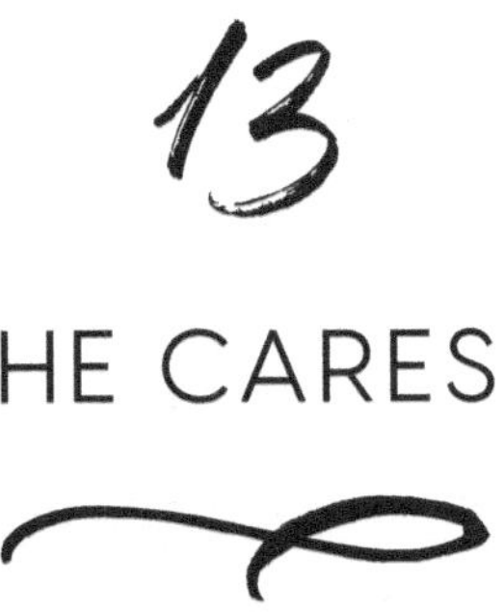

April 29, 2021. I played pickleball again—and I played well! I knew it would be my last game for a while. Little did I know it would be many months before I'd be able to play a full game again. *Lord, give me strength for whatever lies ahead.*

Nurse daughter-in-law Amy called. She had read my reports and a list of the tests ordered from MD. We discussed the upcoming tests, and she assured me she would be available for any conference calls with the doctor. She told me what a wonderful mother-in-law I was. Crying, she choked out this encouragement: "I don't want anything to happen to you. I love you so very much! We are praying when you get here, it will be all gone!"

God has blessed me so with two wonderful daughters-in-law!

More encouraging thoughts and prayers from so many friends. And some even brought gifts: encouragement cards I can give to doctors, nurses, and other cancer patients. Snacks. Lotions, cards, books. Socks and pj's. A prayer book. A devotional book on cancer from a friend who was almost finished with her treatments. She understood what I would be going through. We made plans to study the devotions together long distance each day. Another friend brought a pink cancer bracelet. I felt so blessed to take gifts with me to remind me of these precious friends—and their love and prayers. *Lord, thank you so much for friends and their faith.*

In the evening we went to a Mexican restaurant just down the road from us with Mom and Dad and saw a friend we'd not seen for years. She is about my age. She began to share that she had gone through breast cancer several years before and had been cancer free for five years. I told her about my situation. She shared a lot of things to think about and gave me words of godly encouragement, promising to pray.

Isn't it interesting how God puts people in our paths to encourage us? God's hands would provide protection, guidance, and encouragement to me in the days ahead.

We went home and began preparing for bed. I realized that would be the last night to sleep in my own bed for a while—at least for six weeks of tests and beginning treatments. I was trying hard to relax and rest in peace, knowing God was with me. *Lord, surround our home with angels around every corner of our property. Keep Satan away. Give us strength and healing.*

It was a restless night of wondering. But Scriptures kept running through my mind. And uplifting songs. (You can find the titles to some of these uplifting songs in the song list at the end of this book.)

But the what-ifs continued. God was holding me up, but I could not overcome the fear.

Trust in the Lord. . . .

Reflections

Are you afraid? Afraid of the what-ifs? Afraid of the pain? Afraid of the future? That's so normal. Jesus loves you, and he understands. Keep focusing on him and his love for you.

Casting all your cares [all your anxieties, all your worries, and all your concerns, once and for all] on Him, for He cares about you [with deepest affection, and watches over you very carefully].

— 1 PETER 5:7 AMP

14

GOD IS FIGHTING FOR YOU

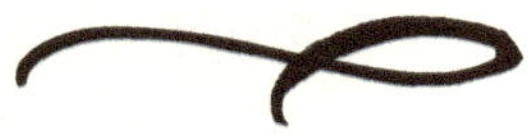

April 30, 2021. Leaving for Texas. Pulling out of the driveway was so overwhelming! I looked at our home we had built together twenty-five years before and the beautiful yard David always kept so well. Tears began streaming down my face. *Will I ever see this home again? Will I ever be able to walk around the yard again? What will happen to our home? Will we have to move somewhere else? Will I die or be in a nursing home? Will we live the rest of our days with our children?*

David looked at me. Seeing the tears and fear, he held my hand and began to pray, asking for peace. I cannot explain how much sadness was in my heart as we drove away.

I can't be the only one who has felt these depressing fears. *Lord, how do people live without your Word, without your strength? Lord, please give me peace. Please protect my home.*

Please care for my parents as I walk this journey. Please keep them well and give them strength as they watch me suffer and fear for me.

We stopped in Dallas for the night. I headed to bed after receiving many texts and prayer assurances.

May 1. We left Dallas and headed toward Amy and Chris's home. When we stopped for a sandwich at a bakery, I noticed a lady wearing a robe and a wig. *Maybe she is having chemo.* She asked me where we were from. We learned she lived just down the road from where we were eating. I told her we were going to see our kids and I was to have breast cancer treatment. She asked my name so she could pray for me.

Another lady was sitting at a table eating. She told us the tomato soup was good, so we got some and headed out. Two hours later we stopped at Buc-ees and ran into that same lady! Recognizing us, she exclaimed, "You just ate at the bakery. I think it's meant for us to meet. Where are you going?" We learned she lived in the Woodlands in Houston. She told us she had a super rare type of lymphoma cancer. Also, three of her friends had just begun breast cancer treatment at MD Anderson. We told her about the deli Chris manages, and she said she would stop by there sometime and ask about me.

I felt as if God was placing angels all around me! I knew the Holy Spirit was guiding me.

As we continued our trip, I received more words of encouragement from friends and family. I needed these daily messages and recorded them in my heart and in my journals.

Reflections

As you walk through your cancer journey, do you feel as if you are in a battle? Ask God to open your eyes so you can see how he is fighting for you. Read how that affected Elisha's servant in 2 Kings 11:11–17.

Look for the blessings every day. See how God is using others to help provide a hedge of protection from the evil one. God will send you prayer warriors to hold you up and encourage you. He will connect you with the right doctors and nurses. He may bring people who have been where you are right now to encourage you. I hope these devotions are part of that!

Writing in my journals helped me so much. If you are not already doing so, I urge you to start writing. Write about your pain and fears and discouragements. But also write about the positive things that are happening. Every positive medical report. The encouragement you are receiving from other people. Those moments when God gives you some special sign that he is with you. And write Scriptures that give you hope and keep you focused on Jesus.

Pleasant words are like a honeycomb, Sweet and delightful to the soul and healing to the body.

— Proverbs 16:24 AMP

15

THAT'S NORMAL

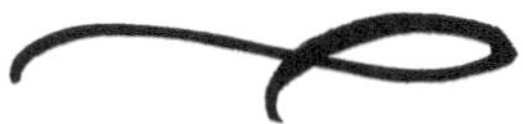

When we arrived at our son's home that evening, Chris said, "Mom, you have been getting mail and gifts all week." I quickly began opening them.

The first was a soft blue and white blanket with encouraging words all over it for the cancer war: *compassion, prayer, positive thoughts, healing energy, peace, love, hope, strength, courage, warrior spirit, radiance,* and *joy*. I determined to take it with me to chemo for comfort in knowing friends were lifting me up in prayer for this battle.

There were so many gifts and cards, it took me several days to open them! I took a picture of each gift as a reminder of who sent it.

Daughter-in-law Amy said, "There are Kleenexes everywhere because I know there will be many tears off and on." I was crying a lot from sadness and fear—and also shedding some happy tears when I thought of the many friends covering me with their love and prayers. This was a very hard emotional journey. At the time, I was not aware these feelings are normal for people recently diagnosed with cancer. I had never walked beside a cancer patient, so I didn't know how difficult it was. I hadn't expected such sadness and fear, but in the months to come, I learned those feelings are normal for cancer patients.

We set out to begin life with Chris and Amy and their children for a yet to be determined length of time. Even though I am sure they were experiencing fear about the future too, they were so supportive and caring to both of us. They had prepared a ground-floor bedroom for us. We were grateful for such a comfortable place to stay and to be with family, but we still had no idea of what lay ahead. Although I was a nurse, I'd never worked with cancer patients. We thought we'd get the treatment plan and then travel back and forth for a while. How wrong we were! The journey would drag on and on with sickness, treatment, surgery, and check-ups.

But God knew. And he had prepared the way.

Reflections

Are you on a cancer journey? If you are plagued with sadness and fear, please understand those feelings are normal for what you are going through. You may be sad about all the things you cannot do right now. Your life has been turned upside down, and you are afraid of what the future may hold. If you have begun treatment, you are probably experiencing all kinds of upsetting side effects.

Understand that those feelings are normal, even for believing Christians. Don't feel guilty. And know that other cancer patients feel the same way.

As much as you can, try to focus on Jesus. Ask him to walk with you through this journey. Trust him for his healing and strength to go through the treatments. Read Scriptures about his faithfulness and his love for you. Here are some to get you started:

Let me hear of your unfailing love each morning, for I am trusting you. Show me where to walk, for I give myself to you.

— PSALM 143:8

Surely God is my help; the Lord is the one who sustains me.

— PSALM 54:4 NIV

Trust in the Lord with all your heart; do not depend on your own understanding. Seek his will in all you do, and he will show you which path to take.

— Proverbs 3:5–6

We know how much God loves us, and we have put our trust in his love. God is love, and all who live in love live in God, and God lives in them.

— 1 John 4:16

— *My Thoughts* —

16

PARTNERSHIPS AND BOUNDARIES

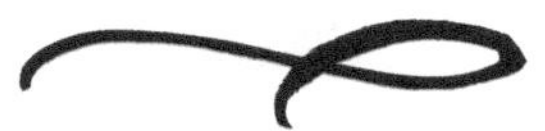

Remember my friend with cancer who gave me a cancer devotional? She and I were reading the same devotional together—day by day. We also prayed together. What a blessing it was to have that kind of mutual understanding and support. I enjoyed the book so much, although I often cried while reading it. I was grateful for other cancer patients willing to talk about their journeys, including their fears and difficult treatments. I pray God will help you and others through this devotional.

Because I realized I would have some hard days, I made rules for the grandchildren about when they could come into my room. I told them they must knock first and wait for Nana or Papa to ask who it is and what they want. Then we would give or deny permission to enter. Once in the room, they were to sit down to play or visit—but no wild jumping or noise because our room was Nana's quiet zone.

May 2, 2021. The children were wonderful. The two oldest, Ava (eleven) and Silas (eight), came into our room that day to say good morning. They asked what I was doing, so I read the verse I was reading at the time: "Thank him for all he has done" (Philippians 4:6). Silas responded, "I remember learning that verse, and it's on my Mimi's wall at her house." They left to get ready for church. Not long after they left, a note from Ava appeared under my door: "Hope you are better."

We went to church, and I was so grateful for fellowship with other believers and the power of the songs and Scriptures—although the tears continued to flow.

After church we went to lunch and then did some shopping. Amy's mom, Judy, who lives close by, came to visit in the evening. The fellowship at dinner and then the playful time with grandkids afterward provided lots of laughs. Although my body and mind seemed to be busy and positive, inside I was still struggling with fear.

Text messages from prayer warriors came throughout the day. It was so important to have people praying for me. I could hear God speaking to me through their messages.

I will endure and God will help me. I must trust him. He loves me, and he will help me. I trust him, and I do not want to be afraid. I call on God. May God stand between me and Satan! Satan, get behind me! I am going to be victorious! We will hold our banner high. God is fighting for me. He will help me defeat this cancer inside me!

I cannot prevent what comes, so Lord, please bring me peace! I am God's child, and I will not allow Satan to steal my joy, for the joy of the Lord is my strength! God knew I was hurting. He knew I had those fears. *I must remain obedient, as Jesus did. He prayed for the cross to pass, but when it didn't, he pressed on as God wanted. I will finish this battle, or I will be with the Lord! But God cares. He holds me—I must trust him.*

Reflections

Do you know another cancer patient who would join you as a prayer partner? Perhaps you could even work through these devotions together. Doing that helped me so much. If not a cancer patient, perhaps a close friend.

So encourage each other and build each other up.

— 1 Thessalonians 5:11

I shared about setting boundaries for my grandchildren. As time went on, I had to do that for friends too. And they understood—in fact, I think they were grateful to know how to help without intruding on time I needed to rest. And how to help me be protected from the possibility of getting sick (especially since COVID was still such a problem at that time). Your loved ones and friends will appreciate your honesty about boundaries.

— *My Thoughts* —

17

PRAYER REMINDERS

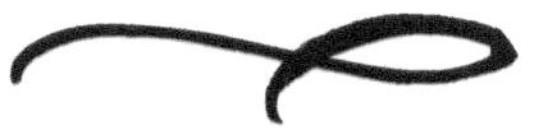

I love Erimish bracelets, so when I was diagnosed with breast cancer, I began giving them to friends as a reminder to pray for me or someone else going through cancer. As time went on, I gave them as a special "thank-you" to medical staff who cared for me and to other cancer patients as a reminder that someone was praying for them. My mother gave them to friends at church to remind them to pray for me.

I printed this message on cards and gave them with the bracelets:

> Erimish bracelets are made in my hometown, Joplin, Missouri. They are the creation of two sisters and entrepreneurs, Ericka and Misha. Their concept was built on empowering women to bring out their own style and share it with the world. The bold and colorful

designs are one-size-fits-most. Erimish jewelry is available in over 10,000 locations, from Nordstrom to local jewelry stores.

> Philippians 4:6 (my paraphrase)
> Do not worry about anything,
> but pray and ask God what you need,
> always giving him thanks.

Many friends and prayer warriors sent me clipart text messages and cards of encouragement. I kept them in my phone notes and read them often during treatments. I recorded them to help me remember the power of prayer and the love of my friends and family. I stored the cards in a box so I could pull them out and reread them when I needed some special encouragement.

It was Sunday evening, and I would officially begin a *long* journey the next day. A journey I had never dreamed I would be taking. One that would need much faith, trust, and positive thinking. I knew I could not lean on my own understanding—only on God's.

> "My thoughts are nothing like your thoughts," says the Lord. "And my ways are far beyond anything you could imagine. For just as the heavens are higher than the earth, so my ways are higher than your ways and my thoughts higher than your thoughts."
>
> — Isaiah 55:8–9

Reflections

I encourage you to consider purchasing or making some sort of prayer reminder to hand out. If you want to consider the Erimish bracelets, you can visit their website at Erimish.com. They make a wonderful thank-you gift as well as a prayer reminder. Your prayer reminder doesn't have to be anything expensive. You may even want to consider customized silicone bracelets with "Pray for [your name]" printed on them.

You are probably receiving some notes and cards. Consider putting them in a special box where you can easily retrieve them to give yourself a lift when you most need it. They will provide the power of God's people lifting you up, people standing in the gap when you feel at your weakest.

My Thoughts

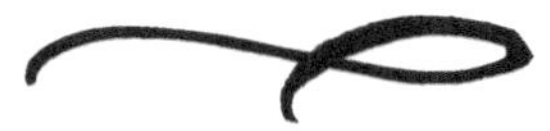

18

NEW EXPERIENCES
BRING NEW FEARS

May 3, 2021. This was it. My first appointment at MD. As I checked in, I learned I was a number—257xxx3. I had to know my number every time I went into the hospital. *I am so glad I am not a number to God. He knows my name . . . my heart . . . how many hairs are on my head! He knows more about me than I know about myself! I am precious to him, and he loves me.*

I reported for my first COVID test, and it was negative. Because the hospital was still under COVID restrictions, the testing center was in the parking lot. Everyone was gowned, masked, and gloved for testing patients. David and Chris had to wait for me all morning in the parking lot.

After the COVID test, I was sent to the main hospital area for additional lab tests. Arriving early, I went right in. As I waited, I looked around—cancer signs everywhere. I felt so alone with David and Chris outside and had a temporary meltdown. Tears began to flow.

On the positive side, I quickly saw a pattern—a wonderful one. Everyone was kind and encouraging. Many even prayed with me. They treated me with love and compassion.

After the tests, Chris, David, and I went to breakfast—it was great! We visited a long time before returning home.

I rested for a while and did some Bible reading, but mostly I cried. Even though I knew God was with me, he had not taken away the cancer. *I have to walk this path God has decided I should take.* I knew he was in control. It was so hard to submit to his control, but who better to be in charge? *I must hold on to my faith!*

Later I went for a walk by myself. Then another walk with Chris. Finally, I walked to Judy's. I talked. She listened. We both cried.

I didn't know all these fears and doubts and tears were a normal part of being a cancer patient. (I learned they are a few weeks later when I attended a support group.)

I must lean on God. His grace will hold me up. He will kill this giant within me just as he enabled David to defeat the giant Goliath. God is fighting for me. He will aim these treatments at the cancer right where it is needed, just as the small rocks David flung from his slingshot hit Goliath in exactly the right spot. (See 1 Samuel 17.)

Reflections

Are you experiencing similar emotions? Sadness. Fear. Do you find yourself crying often? That is so normal for anyone battling cancer. Find someone you can cry with. Someone who will listen to your fears and concerns. Someone who knows when to just sit and listen and seems to know the right thing to say at the right time. Someone who prays with you.

You may experience times when you fear the future. Moments when you wonder if anyone really cares. So many people around me would say the right things, yet they could not understand what I was going through. Their normal life hadn't suddenly come to a halt. My daily life was spent trusting God, talking to him almost every minute, yet walking each day in a fog. Do you feel as if your life is almost over? I did too.

Yes, you will probably have these feelings no matter how strong your faith . . . no matter how long you have been faithful to God . . . no matter if you are a Bible scholar. Each turn you take along the journey will be a new experience that may bring different fears and emotions. Hold on! Strive to be a survivor. Determine to fight this enemy. With Jesus, you can.

Be strong in the Lord [draw your strength from Him and be empowered through your union with Him] and in the power of His [boundless] might.

— EPHESIANS 6:10 AMP

19

PERSISTENT PRAYER

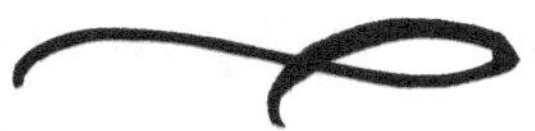

May 4, 2021. No tests scheduled. I was still receiving so many words of encouragement from friends and family. I'd like to share this one with you because it reminded me about the importance of prayer.

> Prayer is so powerful because it joins the hearts of people on earth with the heart of God in heaven. . . . Prayer opens the door for God to work. It is the activity that you and I can engage in on earth when we need the power of heaven to come into our lives and bring wisdom, direction, encouragement, or a miraculous breakthrough. Prayer connects us to the power of God, and that is why it is a greater force than anything else we can ever imagine. . . . Only God's power can bring peace, instill joy, grant wisdom, impart a sense of value and purpose to a

person who doesn't know what to do in life, and work every kind of miracle.[4]

I'm praying for you!

May 5. As I prepared for my appointment, my thoughts were going in every direction. Then these words flowed through my mind: *Be still. Lord, give me wisdom. God, make my mind clear as I ask questions. Lord, please bring me your peace in this war. I am afraid and I have to do this without my family. No one can come with me because of the COVID restrictions.* (David would be waiting in the car for me all day.)

After David kissed me, I walked into the hospital. Again, tears began to flow. I thought about the day I would have to walk alone into heaven. Will there be fear in that walk? No, because I know Jesus will be with me. I believe there will be joy. Oh, to see the face of Jesus and hear his voice.

I found the place for my first test of the day—COVID again. Then they put an armband with my personal number on me. They wanted me to use that number and not my name for the various processing procedures. After signing several papers, I sat down alone for about five minutes before being called into the admissions office. There I met the woman who had kept in touch with me by text and email the previous few weeks. She had gathered all my records and test results from home and set up my first appointments at MD. She was such a blessing. I gave her a Scripture prayer card and a bracelet—and she prayed for me. She was so encouraging as she walked me to the area where I would have a mammogram and ultrasound of my breast.

Reflections

Prayers. Your own prayers. Prayers from friends. From family. From medical personnel. From other cancer patients. So, so important.

Be unceasing and persistent in prayer.

— 1 Thessalonians 5:17 AMP

Now Jesus was telling the disciples a parable to make the point that at all times they ought to pray and not give up and lose heart.

— Luke 18:1 AMP

The heartfelt and persistent prayer of a righteous man (believer) can accomplish much [when put into action and made effective by God—it is dynamic and can have tremendous power].

— James 5:16 AMP

Stay in prayer. Sometimes it may be just one or two words when you are having a treatment or test, but God hears. He sees your heart. And please don't hesitate to ask friends and family to pray for you.

Consider reaching out to a local church or even a cancer organization. There are also online prayer sites and prayer apps. Here are a couple of examples: Pray.com and UpperRoom.org/prayer. This site has other suggestions: margaretfeinberg.com/4-best-prayer-apps-phone.

20

NOT MY WILL, BUT YOURS

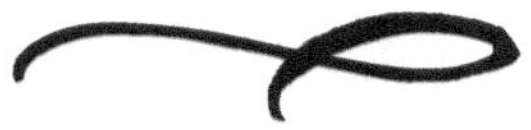

As I mentioned in yesterday's devotions, I was on my way to having a mammogram and ultrasound of my right breast. I was also scheduled for a lymph node biopsy and markers being placed on the spots where the biopsy had been done.

During the mammogram, when the compression of the breast became super painful, I began to get weak and nearly passed out. The women working in the radiology area sat me in a chair and brought me cool washcloths. These ladies were so great!

Then they took me to another room for the ultrasound. A female radiology doctor came in to tell me they needed to do a biopsy of a lymph node. Soon after that biopsy, the lab results came back, confirming cancer. Then she had to put needles back into that area to put another marker so it could be watched throughout the chemo treatments. I almost passed out several times. Again, they sat me down and brought cool cloths. The pain was so bad!

When that was done, the doctor explained that was the only questionable lymph node she had seen, but she wanted to take a biopsy of the left breast as well because there was calcification in the milk glands. I would have to return in a couple of days for that. She cautioned me it would be more painful and last longer. I was not looking forward to that!

When I was thirteen or fourteen, I didn't have any breast development yet, so I stuffed my bra with tissue. Now they want to mash them off? Pain, pain, pain! And to think at fourteen I wanted these boobs? I almost chuckled at the irony.

On this difficult day, I focused a lot on this Scripture:

> We do this by keeping our eyes on Jesus, the champion who initiates and perfects our faith. Because of the joy awaiting him, he endured the cross, disregarding its shame. Now he is seated in the place of honor beside God's throne.

> — HEBREWS 12:2

My mind wandered to the cross in my tree at home. This Scripture was telling me to fix my eyes on Jesus! *I must focus on Jesus and keep trusting in his power! I am sure my pain today was not anything compared with Jesus's pain. All that pain for the sins of man on this earth. For my sins. Oh, Jesus, I am so sorry for all the pain you went through. Thank you for loving me so much.*

Reflections

The night Jesus was arrested, he first went to the Garden of Gethsemane to pray. He began to be sorrowful and troubled, knowing the anguish awaiting him.

"My Father! If it is possible, let this cup of suffering be taken away from me. Yet I want your will to be done, not mine."

— MATTHEW 26:39

He prayed this way three times. We know from these Scriptures that Jesus didn't want the pain. He didn't want to die. He didn't want that horrendous separation from his Father as he took our sins upon him on the cross. But he trusted his Father, and he knew the good that would come from the pain and suffering.

Remember these words of Jesus as you read about my journey and walk through your own valley of sickness. No one wants pain and suffering. We all want to stay on this earth and love our families. To watch them grow. To see them follow the Lord our God with all their hearts, minds, and souls.

If we believe in Jesus and what he did for us . . . if we confess our sins and make him Lord of our life . . . we have the promise of eternal life in heaven, where there are no sorrow, no pain, no tears. We need to trust that he has the best planned for us in heaven. And we need to be willing on this earth to say, "I want your will to be done, not mine."

And we need to believe that even from our own journey of pain and suffering, he will bring good.

And we know that God causes everything to work together for the good of those who love God and are called according to his purpose for them.

— ROMANS 8:28

21

TAKE SOME TIME FOR YOU– AND OTHERS

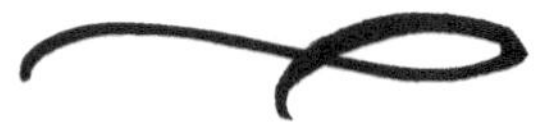

May 6, 2021. Today I must put on the full armor of God. I must let him work. I must wait on him to direct my way!

> Therefore, put on every piece of God's armor so you will be able to resist the enemy in the time of evil. Then after the battle you will still be standing firm. Stand your ground, putting on the belt of truth and the body armor of God's righteousness. For shoes, put on the peace that comes from the Good News so that you will be fully prepared. In addition to all of these, hold up the shield of faith to stop the fiery arrows of the devil. Put on salvation as your helmet, and take the sword of the Spirit, which is the word of God.
>
> — Ephesians 6:13–17

At that time, I did not have joy, but I was trusting in his power and strength through the next rounds of tests.

> We also pray that you will be strengthened with all his glorious power so you will have all the endurance and patience you need. May you be filled with joy, always thanking the Father. He has enabled you to share in the inheritance that belongs to his people, who live in the light.
>
> — Colossians 1:11–12

May 7. More tests. I had to drink lots of water before arriving at the hospital for an early appointment. I was tired—I hadn't slept well because I kept thinking of all the bad things that could happen. *Lord, protect me and give me strength!*

I had a bone scan, a CT scan of my entire body, and an ultrasound of my abdomen. I had to drink a large glass of dye and also received dye through an IV. Because I have a bad reaction to shellfish, I was worried about taking the dye. Some dyes cause reactions similar to that of shellfish. They gave me Benadryl to help prevent reactions—and that made me sleepy. But I knew I would rather be sleepy than not breathing from possible reactions! This was just the beginning of taking Benadryl—I would be taking much more in the following months.

Later that day I received a call about the test results. They showed a tiny cyst on my liver—no cancer was noted, but they would recheck in three months. The doctor said she was sending me a wig prescription through MyChart online. I could get a wig whenever I was ready. She also sent five prescriptions for me to take after the first chemo treatment.

May 8. Saturday. Judy and I went to dinner and to an outside concert. The setting was beautiful—and very relaxing. We had dinner at a cute restaurant. The food was good, and I enjoyed the outing so much.

Reflections

Although your activity may be limited while you go through testing and treatment, I encourage you to take some time for yourself. Outings like this one with Judy helped me get my mind off the problems and just relax and enjoy a few hours. When possible, do fun things with friends you enjoy. Laughter makes it even better. "A cheerful heart is good medicine" (Proverbs 17:22).

When cancer tests and treatments aren't the center of your life, find positive ways to fill the time. Ask God for direction! Some things I focused on included praying for others . . . finding ways to encourage others . . . and serving others with food and love. You may focus on friends or family in need. You are probably meeting other cancer patients. Consider reaching out to them.

Think about the ways others are blessing you. Think about the ways God is comforting you. That will spark ideas about how you can help others.

We've looked at these verses before, but it's good to meditate on them often.

All praise to God, the Father of our Lord Jesus Christ. God is our merciful Father and the source of all comfort. He comforts us in all our troubles so that we can comfort others. When they are troubled, we will be able to give them the same comfort God has given us.

— 2 Corinthians 1:3–4

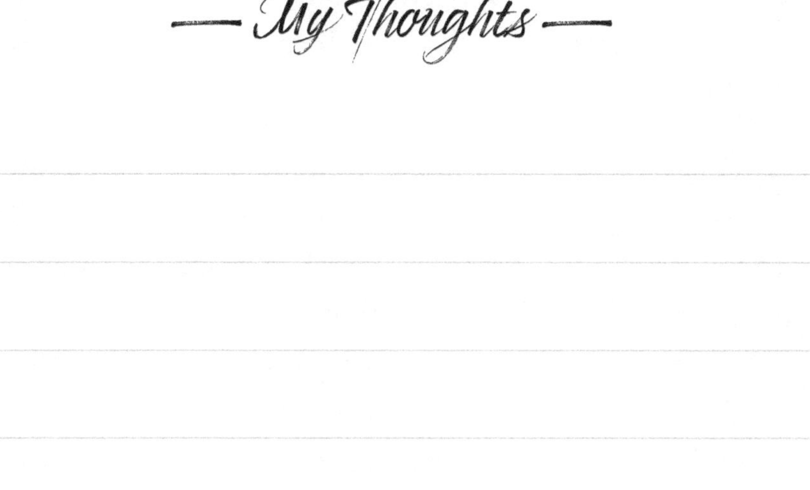

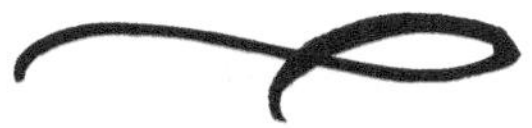

FOCUS ON THE POSITIVES

May 9, 2021. Mother's Day! I was so blessed to be with family on this special occasion. We went to church and then out for a great meal. In the afternoon, Amy, Ava, Judy, and I went to get manicures. Then we had so much fun at a circus and acrobat show in the evening. What a delightful day! God was showing me ways to enjoy life even during that difficult time.

I received several gifts, including flowers and strawberries from David. Some of the presents were "C" gifts, including a pink cancer watchband. Although I was not excited about this new part of my life, the gifts were super! *Thank you, Lord, for the creative gifts people are sending me to help bring me happiness as I walk these new steps in my life. Lord, please take out the "C." Heal me so I can say my ~~cancer~~ is gone by the power of God!* (At MD Anderson ~~Cancer~~ Center, *cancer* is always marked out on their signs and papers.)

May 10. I saw my surgeon. I would see her every two to three months during chemo so she could monitor the cancer. I learned I would have surgery at the main hospital in downtown Houston three to four weeks after completing chemo. After the surgery, I would have a one-night hospital stay. Three to four weeks post-op, I would return to see my surgeon.

She explained I would have two drains on each side if I had a double mastectomy. At that time, she didn't think a double mastectomy would be needed. In fact, depending on how the tumor responded to the chemo, she said they may do only a lumpectomy. I would have post-op radiation, but we wouldn't know how many treatments until after surgery since that would depend on how many lymph nodes were affected.

She also explained I would have another fourteen rounds of chemo after surgery! A full year of treatment. David and I had a special trip planned. She said not to cancel until we saw how treatments went and the time frame of my surgery.

I learned that when cancer is in a lymph node, chemo is done before surgery in hope of killing it. Since I had one node with cancer, I would begin with chemo—six rounds of four drugs. The doctor did not see cancer in any other organs. That was a praise for me! I tried hard to focus on these positive reports.

Reflections

I knew I had to focus on every positive report and word of encouragement to keep from drowning in the pain and fear. I encourage you to do that too.

Don't worry about anything; instead, pray about everything. Tell God what you need, and thank him for all he has done. Then you will experience God's peace, which exceeds anything we can understand. His peace will guard your hearts and minds as you live in Christ Jesus. And now, dear brothers and sisters, one final thing. Fix your thoughts on what is true, and honorable, and right, and pure, and lovely, and admirable. Think about things that are excellent and worthy of praise. Keep putting into practice all you learned and received from me—everything you heard from me and saw me doing. Then the God of peace will be with you.

— Philippians 4:6–9

My Thoughts

23

LEAN ON HIM

Trust in the Lord with all your heart; do not depend on your own understanding. Seek his will in all you do, and he will show you which path to take.

— Proverbs 3:5–6

This verse went over and over in my mind as I listened to the doctor explaining about the chemo drugs they planned to give me. Some were called Red Devil drugs— later I would understand why. They took me right to the door of hell and made me fear death. The side effects made me weak and sick. I was confused and not able to think clearly. Later I learned that these drugs cause "chemo brain."

Oh, Lord. I know medicines, and I understand many things about the body, but I cannot lean on my own understanding now. You know more about my body than I do. Day by day, hour by hour, please show me which paths to take. Please protect me through this treatment.

I would be given six rounds of four drugs every three weeks, along with several medications before each infusion to help prevent side effects. I would also take medicines for five to ten days following the chemo to further reduce reactions. The medications before each chemo treatment would make me very sleepy. The medical team would pack my feet and hands in ice while one of the drugs was infusing to help decrease, but not prevent, neuropathy and nerve damage.

They gave me a list of the drugs I would take during and after each chemo infusion and another list of over-the-counter meds to help with side effects. Whew! These were long lists.

Probable side effects included watering eyes, vision problems, numbness in feet and hands, and hair loss. The treatments would lower potassium, iron, and magnesium levels. There would also be diarrhea, heart problems, rashes, and sores and a metal taste in my mouth.

This was so overwhelming. I had taken very few medicines throughout my life—mostly only if I had the flu or a cold and when I had COVID. Now I needed a spreadsheet to figure out what I should take and when. I was becoming a druggie!

Lord, please protect my body! Lord, hear my cry! I am panicking again. Just thinking about these drugs is filling me with fear. Lord, keep my spirit calm, and do not let my spirit give way to fear. Please help me be strong. God, come to save me and cause my body to rebuild from the chemo.

Reflections

I am not sharing these details to frighten you. If you've not yet begun chemo treatment, I hope this information will help you be more prepared for discussing all this with your doctor, for the lists of medicines, and for the side effects that will most likely follow.

Whether this part is yet to come for you or you are in the midst of it or it's behind you, I want you to know that the fear you may experience is normal. But remember, you are never, ever alone. Jesus is holding your hand. He will be with you every moment. Don't even try to understand what you are experiencing—instead, trust him. Seek his will and his plan above all else. He will show you, step-by-step, what to do. Again, meditate on Isaiah 41:10.

"Don't be afraid, for I am with you. Don't be discouraged, for I am your God. I will strengthen you and help you. I will hold you up with my victorious right hand."

24

DIET AND EXERCISE

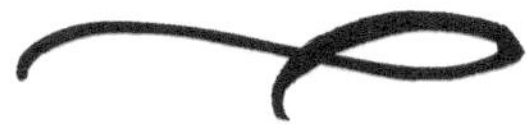

A video conference with a cancer dietary nurse helped me begin to plan a healthy diet for my journey. She said a plant-based diet is best. I was to focus on drinking seventy ounces of Core water and eating fruit, greens, and meats daily. Breads should be grains, nuts, or seeds. She recommended Dave's Killer Bread or any kind of sourdough. I was to eat low-fiber breads—no more than two grains of fiber per slice. I couldn't eat butter because it upset my stomach. I was not to eat more than thirty grams of protein per meal. Nuts were good to eat. And she said the best milk was Silk.

As I considered all this, these Scriptures came to mind.

"And don't be concerned about what to eat and what to drink. Don't worry about such things. . . . Your Father already knows your needs."

— Luke 12:29–30

"Look at the birds. They don't plant or harvest or store food in barns, for your heavenly Father feeds them. And aren't you far more valuable to him than they are?"

— Matthew 6:26

I knew God would help me eat correctly. Even the birds don't worry about what they will eat!

The doctors told me that during treatment, chemo patients usually end up in the hospital several times with dehydration and low blood counts. *Lord, please hold me up as you do the birds of the air! Lord, walk with me. I pray I won't have so many side effects that I have to be in the hospital during treatment. Lord, please do not leave me alone in this battle!*

The dietitian and doctors encouraged me to nap for two hours each afternoon to allow my body to rest and rebuild. They recommended daily meditation—I focused on God's Word. Regular exercise and deep breathing to relax were also recommended.

This journey was not going to be easy for me. *God, why? Why did you allow this to come into my life?* I couldn't understand why God had allowed this but remembered I needed to lean on his understanding, not mine. Every day many Scriptures came to me and provided me with strength for each moment.

Reflections

The dietary plan your medical team recommends may seem overwhelming, but remember that God is with you and will help. "Your Father already knows your needs." Take time to read the Bible every day, no matter how rough you are feeling.

But those who trust in the Lord will find new strength. They will soar high on wings like eagles. They will run and not grow weary. They will walk and not faint.

— Isaiah 40:31

Depending on your doctor's instructions, you may want to exercise regularly. I did but was careful not to overdo with heavy weights or extended times of working out. I spaced my exercise out over the day. That was hard for me as I had been working out with weights and walking regularly for years. I missed my daily one to three hours playing pickleball.

The right diet and exercise won't eliminate all the side effects of treatment—but they can sure help.

The most important part of all is to keep your eyes on Jesus. Trust him. Trust his love. Trust him to stay with you. And trust his plan.

Wait for the Lord; be strong and take heart and wait for the Lord.

— Psalm 27:14 NIV

25

RUNNING THE RACE

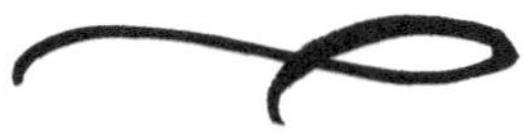

May 10, 2021. I received this note from my mom: "You are the prized and precious child of God. Pour out your heart to him and tell him your needs. He is always open to you."

> The Lord hears his people when they call to him for help. He rescues them from all their troubles. The Lord is close to the brokenhearted; he rescues those whose spirits are crushed.
>
> — PSALM 34:17–18

May 11. My heart doctor did an echo, an EKG, an aorta scan, and an ultrasound of my heart. Amy works with this doctor, so she came to the appointment with David and me.

The doctor's first words to me were, "How is your spirit?"

My reply? "How would anyone's spirit feel with just getting a cancer diagnosis and living with my children for an unknown time?"

He responded sweetly, "So how is your spirit? Your faith?"

"Oh, my faith! Well, I believe if God wants me to live, I will live. And if I die today, I know I will go to heaven. I believe in God!"

He answered with confidence. "Then you will make it through this. Your tests are perfect. You do have a slight left center valve leak, but you have a very strong heart for a seventy-year-old. You should do well through chemo."

I jumped off the bed and danced around the room. "Praise the Lord. Praise the Lord. Finally, a perfect test! Oh, thank you, Lord." Tears streamed down my cheeks—this time, tears of joy and thanksgiving.

When I settled down a bit, the doctor continued. "These drugs may cause heart problems, so we will check it every three months until a few months following your last treatment in about two years." He gave me a prescription for high blood pressure to take as needed if I should get overanxious before a treatment or have an elevated pressure from the chemo.

My next appointment that day was a video Zoom with an anesthesiologist for my upcoming port placement surgery. It would be that week, so chemo could begin as soon as possible.

Reflections

I hope you are taking every opportunity to praise God and rejoice. With so many negative things going on, it becomes more important than ever to rejoice about the good and give God the glory. I may have looked a little silly dancing around the doctor's office, but I knew everyone watching was rejoicing with me. And, most important, God heard me.

Then I will praise God's name with singing, and I will honor him with thanksgiving.

— Psalm 69:30

We were able to record our doctors' visits. If you are not doing that, consider asking for permission so you can review them later. I often didn't remember everything they said—there was so much information, combined with my fear and anxiety. I found it a blessing to be able to play it back for myself—and for family. Sometimes I listened to the recordings even months later to remind myself of test results and what treatment was coming next.

Several of the doctors told me, "Your personal belief plays a major role in healing you physically. Keep your mind positive!" They encouraged me to keep my faith in God and his power. And David told me often, "We can do this. We will get through it! You will be well someday. God's hand is healing you and providing strength and power in protecting you from more sickness!"

God will do that for you too. Keep your eyes on him. Be determined to run the race set before you—with him.

Let us run with endurance the race God has set before us. We do this by keeping our eyes on Jesus, the champion who initiates and perfects our faith.

— HEBREWS 12:1–2

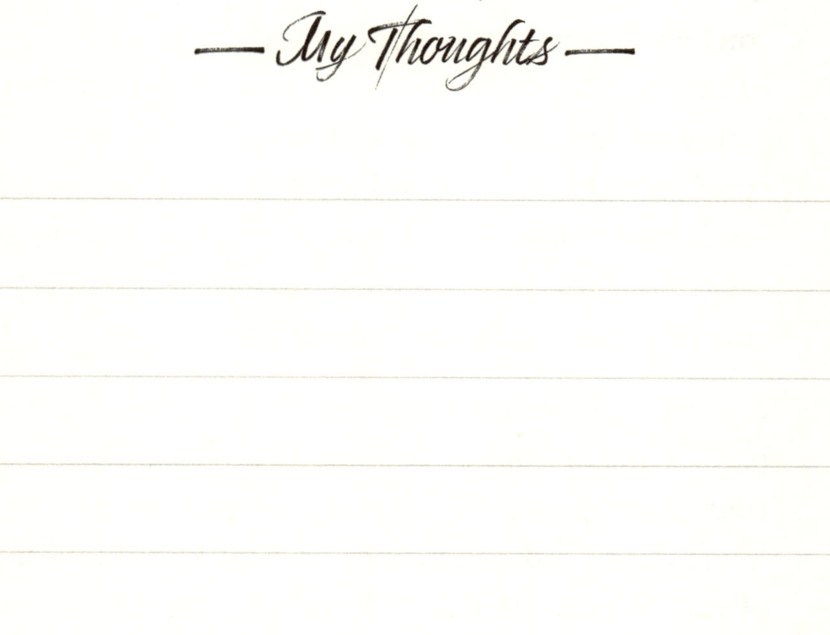

26

EYES ON JESUS, NOT THE WAVES

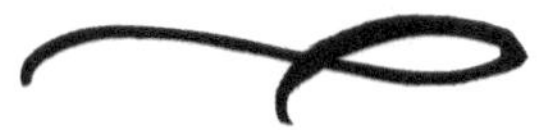

May 12, 2021. I had a left breast stereotactic biopsy. Very, very painful. It was done with large needles while my breast was kept compressed in the mammogram machine. They left the needles in place to take pictures and then moved them again and again. To position the needles correctly, they took X-rays. My breast remained compressed until they retrieved all the tissue needed for biopsy. The lab staff stood by to take the tissue for testing as soon as possible.

To get through this test, I reminded myself of Peter and Jesus walking on the water. The disciples were crossing the lake in the midst of a storm. They looked up and saw Jesus walking on the water toward them.

Then Peter called to him, "Lord, if it's really you, tell me to come to you, walking on the water." "Yes, come," Jesus said. So Peter went over the side of the boat and walked on the water toward Jesus. But when he saw the strong wind and the waves, he was terrified and began to sink. "Save me, Lord!" he shouted. Jesus immediately reached out and grabbed him. "You have so little faith," Jesus said. "Why did you doubt me?" When they climbed back into the boat, the wind stopped. Then the disciples worshiped him. "You really are the Son of God!" they exclaimed.

— MATTHEW 14:28–33

When Peter kept his eyes on Jesus, he was fine. But then he took his eyes off Jesus and focused on the raging waves all around him—and he began to sink.

I thought about this and just before the procedure found a spot on the wall and pictured it as Jesus's face. I trusted he would not let me sink. I would not take my eyes off his face. I did not want to drown. Jesus was my strength. I knew he would hold me up!

A couple of times the nurse said, "We need to move you just a little." Each time I responded, "Don't move me till I find another spot to see Jesus." I had to keep my eyes on him. The staff were understanding and acknowledged Jesus would help me get through it. The test took a long time, and I became weak and faint, but as I kept my eyes on Jesus, I made it to the end!

Reflections

I urge you to find a way to keep your eyes on Jesus when you are enduring painful tests. When we focus on the waves, as Peter did, we begin to sink. Focus on Jesus. Know he is there with you, holding your hand.

"Don't be afraid, for I am with you. Don't be discouraged, for I am your God. I will strengthen you and help you. I will hold you up with my victorious right hand."

— Isaiah 41:10

God will carry you through. You may not know how, but trust that he will. I knew Satan was looking for those moments I felt the weakest to attempt to make me fearful. I spoke these words: "Get behind me, Satan. Jesus's blood is all over me, and you can't get through!" Satan could not steal my joy unless I allowed him to. The same is true for you. Stay focused on Jesus, on his promises, and on his love and power. Keep pressing on.

The one who is in you [Jesus] is greater than the one who is in the world [Satan].

— 1 John 4:4 NIV

27

SHHH . . .
GOD IS IN CONTROL

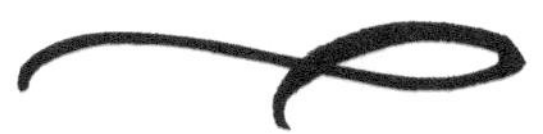

Following the biopsy, I went to a surgery area on the third floor for my port placement. Because of COVID restrictions, no one could go with me. Fear began to overtake me while I was on the elevator, and tears streamed down my cheeks. Immediately I began to speak Scripture and ask God for strength. And I remembered—his mighty hand was holding me. I reminded myself to cling to my faith. And I remembered these people were trained nurses and doctors, and they didn't want anything to go wrong.

After arriving in the surgery area, I was given several drugs that made me sleepy. The doctor said if I didn't lie very still, they would need to put me completely to sleep. Not wanting that, I determined to lie there without moving. To do that, I couldn't even talk. I am a very talky person, so that was hard!

It took about an hour for them to insert the port in my left shoulder, with a thirteen-inch catheter going into my neck and down into my heart. The incision was about three inches long on my left upper chest area.

A short time after the procedure was finished, they called David to come to the door, and then they took me to the car in a wheelchair. I had ice packs on my breast, an ace wrap around my chest, and bandages on my left shoulder where they had placed the port.

I had not been able to drink or eat anything since the previous night at midnight and was hungry from all those hours of fasting. And I was emotional. *This is real. This is cancer!*

Thursday, Friday, and Saturday were days of rest and light activity. I walked two miles every day and went wig shopping with Judy. One evening she and I went to a concert at a small restaurant. All this helped keep my mind on things other than cancer, but occasionally the fear and pain slipped through, and tears fell.

During that time, I considered this verse:

> He who began a good work in you will carry it on to completion.

> — PHILIPPIANS 1:6 NIV

What does that mean? Do I have more work to do on earth? Or is God almost finished with me here? Whatever the answer to those questions, I knew God was in control. And he was definitely the best one to be in control. I knew he loved me and had a plan. He had always known this time would come. Even though I was going through so much pain and I wasn't sure what the outcome would be, I knew we are promised eternal life with God after we leave this world. *This is so hard to do, but I know God will provide me with whatever I need to take this journey.*

Reflections

No matter what happens during your cancer journey, remember you are not alone. God will give you the power and strength you need. He will get you through the tests, biopsies, chemo, scans, surgery, radiation—whatever comes. As you fix your eyes on Jesus, he will calm you . . . strengthen you . . . and help you.

Say this: "I am God's child, and I will not allow Satan to steal my joy. I will fix my eyes on Jesus. My hope is in him. I will not be afraid."

"I am leaving you with a gift—peace of mind and heart. And the peace I give is a gift the world cannot give. So don't be troubled or afraid."

— JOHN 14:27

— My Thoughts —

28

SPECIAL MOMENTS
FROM GOD

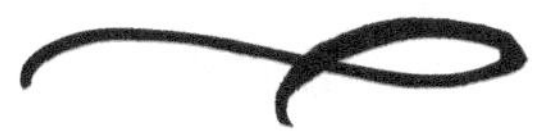

May 16, 2021. It was Sunday, and we went to church. Hurting from all the bruises and cuts to my breast and body, I had been using ice packs and taking Tylenol. I couldn't sleep in any position except on my back. Everything hurt in my chest area.

In the late afternoon, Chris said he had someplace to go. Returning later, he called me from my room. "Mom, come here!" To my surprise, there stood our son Shon from North Carolina! I was so happy to see him, I cried and cried. I knew he was there for my first chemo that week.

Our Bible study small group FaceTimed me to pray for my strength. It was a blessing to have some prayer warriors see me with hair. It would soon be gone for many months. Their hands were holding me up to God!

I received another note from my mom: "The Lord allows problems and trials to build us up. God wants us to seek him and rely on his strength. His heart and his throne room are always open to you. 'But when I am afraid, I will put my trust in you.' (Psalm 56:3). In God I trust, and I am not afraid. God goes with you."

A minister for the cancer support group at Chris's church came to pray for me. He brought me a small wooden cross to carry to each chemo treatment. I kept the cross with me through all the treatments. It was a strong bond to Jesus! Remember the cross in the tree in my backyard?

That was a sad hair day. I asked Amy's hairdresser to come to the house and shave my hair. I knew I'd lose my hair from chemo and didn't want to watch it come out each day on my bed pillow. As she was cutting, Amy and Judy cried. I prayed quietly, asking God for strength, and reminded myself it was only hair. But being bald was not easy. I knew my looks would change from that day forward.

When she finished, they put all my hair into a ziplock bag for me to keep. I don't think I've ever looked at it again!

We took pictures of David and me, and then of me with the various family members. I looked strong. I was smiling, but in my heart, I felt fear, pain, and sadness. *Oh, Lord, please walk with me!*

He will cover you with his feathers, and under his wings you will find refuge.

— PSALM 91:4 NIV

Lord, please cover this bald head. Bring me peace.

Reflections

Even during this difficult day, God blessed me in so many ways. Attending the church service. Being surrounded by family during the day. Shon arriving unexpectedly. My friends praying for me on FaceTime. Receiving the precious and encouraging note from my mom. The minister praying for me and giving me the cross. And having someone who was willing to come to the house to cut my hair.

Even during your most difficult times, I encourage you to look for the positive. See God's hand at work. Remember he loves you. And thank him.

But as for me, I will sing about your power. Each morning I will sing with joy about your unfailing love. For you have been my refuge, a place of safety when I am in distress.

— PSALM 59:16

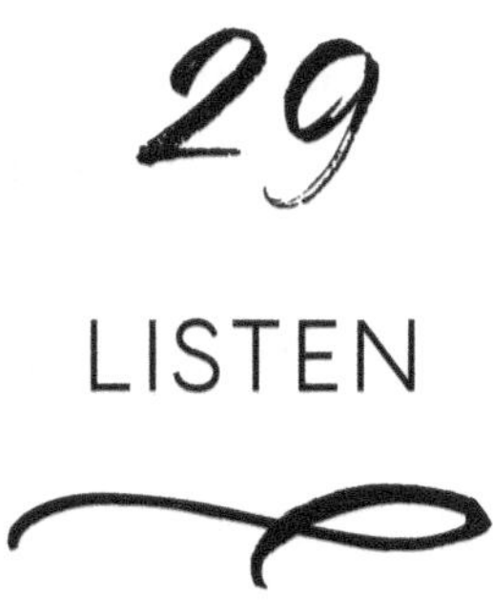

LISTEN

May 17, 2021. The next day chemo would begin. In the early evening I was sitting in my room, still sad about my hair. My bald head was cold. Suddenly, my grandson Sawyer rushed in. "Hurry, Nana! Come see the colors—a rainbow!"

I stepped outside to see not only a rainbow—but a double rainbow! Sawyer was so excited. "It's a big rainbow—orange, green, pink! It's big, big, big. It's a great big one!"

I was excited too. I believed God was reassuring me he would be with me as he was with Noah. When God shut the ark door, I am sure Noah experienced fear and wonder about what would happen to his family. As he rode in that boat all those months, he must have wondered if he would ever get out alive. He may have even been injured from a rough ride. The animals may have been hard to handle. Think of the smell! And so much work to feed all those creatures every day.

Without light from outside, it may have been dark most of the day. Perhaps he experienced times of fear. Times of asking God *why*. But he had been faithful to obey God by building the ark over a period of many years. Although he had been continually being ridiculed by all the people, he had obeyed. And he remained faithful during all that time on the ark. He may have asked God when the journey would be over, but he seemed to trust the Lord, no matter what.

Then as he stepped out of the boat many months later, there was a rainbow!

> And God said, "This is the sign of the covenant I am making between me and you and every living creature with you, a covenant for all generations to come: I have set my rainbow in the clouds, and it will be the sign of the covenant between me and the earth. Whenever I bring clouds over the earth and the rainbow appears in the clouds, I will remember my covenant between me and you and all living creatures of every kind. Never again will the waters become a flood to destroy all life. Whenever the rainbow appears in the clouds, I will see it and remember the everlasting covenant between God and all living creatures of every kind on the earth."
>
> — GENESIS 9:12–16 NIV

That day I realized God was promising me he is faithful and would carry me through to the end! I believed he was promising me I would ride out the storm, and everything would be okay.

Lord, I know you will hold me up and walk with me. Thank you for reminding me of your power over the earth and your power over me and my life. I still have so much fear of the unknown. This journey will be a rough ride. Hold me, Lord!

God had given me precious reassurance the night before chemo began.

Reflections

Is the ride on your journey rough right now? Listen for God's voice. It may be a still, small voice like the one Elijah heard (1 Kings 19). Or it may be something as visible as a rainbow or a cross in a tree. It may be through a Bible passage that jumps out at you . . . or through the words of a friend. The possibilities are limitless. But he is speaking. He wants to encourage you. Learn to listen, even through the pain.

"My sheep listen to my voice."

— JOHN 10:27

My Thoughts

30

NEVER ALONE

Maay 18, 2021. This was the day of my first chemo treatment. COVID restrictions were still in effect, so I had to enter the hospital alone, saying goodbye to David and our sons, Shon and Chris, as I walked through the door. They would wait in the parking lot for me.

My first stop was at the lab for blood work. Then I saw the doctor and learned the biopsy of my left breast showed no cancer! However, it did show some calcification in the milk glands, which would have to be watched. The cancer in my right breast had begun from calcification in the milk glands. When the pickleball had hit my breast, the milk gland had broken open and allowed room for the aggressive cancer to grow.

My blood work came back normal, and I was cleared for the chemo treatment. First, I gave the doctor and her nurses each a bracelet and asked them to continue praying for me. They were so pleased and promised to pray.

Then I went to the chemo infusion room. I felt so alone but then focused on the fact that even if my family couldn't be with me, God was there. *Lord, hold my hand, and take care of me.*

First, I received pre-med IVs to help with side effects. Then, over the next eight minutes, they gave me two drugs just under the skin on my left thigh. A large bubble of fluid formed in my skin tissue. It would slowly absorb over the next few days but was very sore.

The nurse dressed in gowns, gloves, a mask, and a hair covering to prevent her from being exposed to the Red Devil chemo drugs they would be putting in my veins. Really?

Lord, give me strength to get through this. I pray there will be no side effects I can't handle.

The nurse started the infusion with the first drug. It took about ninety minutes. Afterward, she flushed my port with saline. Then she did the same protective dress routine and returned with the next bag of chemo drugs, which infused for about an hour. After that, the port was flushed out with more blood-thinning medicine and saline. I was very drowsy from some of the pre-meds, including Benadryl.

Reflections

I hope a friend or family member will be able to accompany you to your infusions. But even if you are sometimes alone, remember you are not really alone.

For God has said, "I will never fail you. I will never abandon you."

— HEBREWS 13:5

When I was about to begin the chemo treatments, Amy helped me set up a site on CaringBridge. It's a website where you can share updates about your medical journey to friends around the world. Their website (www.caringbridge.org) describes it this way:

CaringBridge is your free online tool for sharing health updates. It is an easy and ad-free way to communicate health news to family and friends—all in one place.[5]

It's very easy to sign up. You can post as often as you like, and friends and family can respond to your posts. They also have a planner you can use to help you manage your to-do list, which has probably become rather overwhelming at this point.

My posts were simplified stories of my journey. You can post daily. I chose to post just every few weeks, summarizing what I'd written in my journal. If you don't feel up to doing your own posts, you can add someone close to you as a coauthor. I hope you will check it out. It's a wonderful way to stay in touch and keep all your prayer warriors and loved ones up-to-date with one post instead of many texts, emails, or phone calls.

— *My Thoughts* —

31

FIX YOUR THOUGHTS . . .

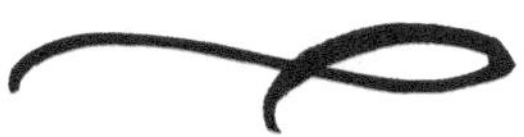

After the chemo treatment, the team explained that my blood count would drop over the following twenty-four to forty-eight hours. To help build it back up, they put medicine in a little box called an on-body injector (OBI). It would automatically inject a blood-builder medicine into my body in twenty-seven hours. After double-taping the box on the left side of my abdomen, they pressed the button on the box. After fifteen seconds of beeping, suddenly a needle went into my abdomen. It was like a gunshot invading my body! I learned the needle had just placed a small catheter inside me.

This small machine could not be exposed to sunlight. It could not be any closer than four to six inches to a cell phone, electrical equipment, cordless phones, microwaves, or appliances—they would interfere with the countdown and performance. It could not be exposed to MRI, X-ray, CT, ultrasound, or oxygen environments.

They cautioned me to wear loose clothing so the box wouldn't get pulled off. I could not shower or soak in a tub because it had to be kept dry. I couldn't lie on it and risk dislodging the small catheter.

While activated, the small box had a green light that flashed every few seconds. I felt like a lightning bug! After twenty-seven hours, when it was ready to inject, it would flash more quickly and beep. Then it would inject the medicine over a period of forty-five minutes. When the injection was finished, the light would become solid green, and the top of the box would say "empty." Then we could remove it, making sure the small catheter remained on the box and the entire area was dry. If at any time during the process, the light turned red or we saw fluid leaking, we were to call the hospital emergency care team and keep the device so they could examine it.

I was finally ready to leave the hospital. I was so thankful for the chemo team. Nurses who spoke of God offered encouraging words, focusing on everything positive that had happened. I also received peace from text messages, uplifting Scriptures, and music playing on my phone all day. Songs of God fighting the battle.

To top it all off, as I came out the hospital doors mid-afternoon, there stood three handsome men smiling at me. I don't think I'd ever been happier to see my husband and sons. I shed tears of joy and gratitude, knowing they had been praying for me as they waited.

Reflections

As you go through treatments, I encourage you to find positive things to focus on. You may want to take your Bible with you . . . or you may find it more helpful to write out some of your favorite verses on index cards. Meditate on them . . . read them aloud . . . pray them.

I also found comfort in playing some encouraging music on my phone throughout the treatment. (Some of my favorites are listed at the end of this book.) You may want to prepare a playlist of songs that lift you up and help you keep your eyes on Jesus throughout the battle.

If a friend or loved one is with you, talk about positive things. Part of the time, you may want to encourage each other in the Lord. Maybe spend some time laughing about funny and happy memories. And definitely talk about things you plan to do in the future!

Fix your thoughts on what is true, and honorable, and right, and pure, and lovely, and admirable. Think about things that are excellent and worthy of praise.

— PHILIPPIANS 4:8

— *My Thoughts* —

32

SIDE EFFECTS BEGIN

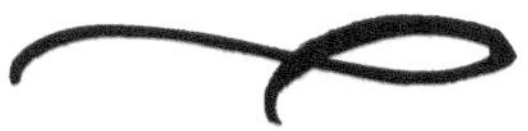

May 19, 2021. The day following my first chemo treatment, I walked about two miles around the neighborhood with Shon. He was scheduled to leave for home the next day. I was so thankful he had come to be with me for my first chemo treatment. He is a faithful praying man, and his encouragement meant so much.

I was feeling well enough later in the day for Judy and me to go get a wig from a ministry that supplies them for cancer patients. They also have counselors, exercise classes, support groups, and social events. They gave me my first wig free! What a wonderful ministry! Then we went to lunch and to Dillard's for some shoes.

I was ready for a nap. We went home, and I slept for two hours. Then, exactly twenty-seven hours after they had put the OBI on me, it went off. After it finished injecting the medicine, the light went from flashing green to solid green and then said "empty." Amy helped me remove it with no problems. They had explained that the injected drug would help rejuvenate blood cells, bringing some bone pain in about four days.

I didn't eat much for dinner, and as the day wore on, I was not feeling well. I took some meds to help prevent nausea and pain. After visiting with the family for a while, I went to bed about eleven o'clock.

May 20. About 5:30 in the evening, I wasn't feeling well at all and tried to reach the doctor on call, but the number wasn't working. I was developing a raspy voice and having some difficulty breathing. My face and neck were very red, and taking another Benadryl didn't seem to help. I decided to go to the Methodist hospital ER where Amy worked. She met us in the ER, and I was taken to a room quickly. My vitals were fine. They did some labs and gave me IV fluids (Pepcid and Benadryl) and a steroid. When breathing became less difficult, they dismissed me for home just after midnight. Everyone was so wonderful to me!

As the ER team had suggested, I took Benadryl, Claritin, and Zofran after getting home. Then I began having liquid yellow diarrhea and took some Imodium. The diarrhea stopped about four in the morning. Throughout the night, I had a tingling sensation all over my body, accompanied by chills and shaking.

Lord, now I am even more afraid of reactions to the drugs I will be taking for months. Please give me the courage and strength. Help me focus on you!

Reflections

Your side effects may differ from mine. However, I want to share these details of my experience—not to frighten you but to help you be prepared and understand that side effects are normal. And the fear that comes is normal as well. But more importantly, I want to encourage you to remember that Jesus is with you every second. Turn to him. Lean on him. Trust him. He loves you and is holding your hand.

I found so much rest in this Scripture:

God is our refuge and strength, always ready to help in times of trouble. So we will not fear when earthquakes come and the mountains crumble into the sea. Let the oceans roar and foam. Let the mountains tremble as the waters surge!

— Psalm 46:1–3

I knew no matter what came, God would be with me. He is with you too—no matter what.

My Thoughts

33

HIS WAY . . . HIS STRENGTH

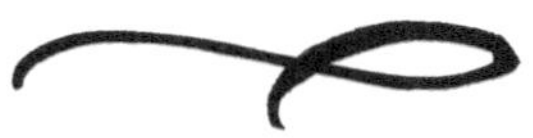

May 21, 2021. In the morning, my neck was still red, face slightly swollen, and my voice still a bit raspy. I weighed myself to find I had gained three and a half pounds since the chemo treatment. I texted the doctor in MyChart to describe the symptoms and ER visit. I sent her pictures of my face, the arm rash, and the IV port. Her nurse responded later that day saying that the rash seemed to be fading and the port looked good. After making several adjustments to my meds, she cautioned that if the rash worsened or I had any trouble breathing to return to the ER.

May 22. I was feeling better, but the doctor called to encourage me to take it easy and rest often because I may experience extreme fatigue for about a week.

As of that day, we had been in Texas over three weeks. Because we did not know how I would react to any of the treatments, my medical team wanted us to stay close to MD Anderson, especially since I did not have an oncologist at home yet.

I would be getting chemo every three weeks, a total of six rounds—the next one on June 8. Following these treatments would come the breast surgery. After that healed, I would have six weeks of radiation. We planned for David to return home at some point to take care of things around the house and then return to Texas. I hoped I would be able to go home for a short stay sometime during the chemo.

That evening I became nervous and began crying. Diarrhea and nausea persisted, and I felt faint. Amy gave me more of the anti-nausea medicine. When that took effect, I was able to go to bed.

I let my friends and family know that I may not be able to respond to text messages or calls because of sickness, emotional struggles, or busy treatment schedules. I explained about CaringBridge and that when I wasn't up to posting, family members would do updates for me there and friends could respond. I appreciated all their care and concern so much. I was often reminded of the faithful friends in the story of the paralytic in Luke 5:17–26 who believed in Jesus so strongly and loved their friend so much that they got through the crowds around Jesus by lowering him through the roof! My friends were like that, and what a difference they made during this journey.

Even with all the encouragement and love, during this time I was repeatedly gripped with fear. I knew God had me in his all-powerful, all-loving hands, but I struggled to trust him. I was so accustomed to being a strong person, but now I needed to lean completely on his strength. I knew I shouldn't be afraid or sad or cry so much, but it was so hard. I rested in his Word. *God, remove Satan from around me and bring me hope!*

Reflections

If you are like me, you have at least a little "I can do it myself" in you! I think one of the good things God brings from our difficult times is that we become more aware of our dependence on him. He doesn't want us to do things in our own strength—or in our own way. Why? Because he loves us and knows that only when we trust him completely can he help us the way he wants to. His plan. His timing. His understanding. His strength. So much better than ours!

Trust in the Lord with all your heart; do not depend on your own understanding. Seek his will in all you do, and he will show you which path to take. Don't be impressed with your own wisdom. Instead, fear the Lord and turn away from evil. Then you will have healing for your body and strength for your bones.

— Proverbs 3:5–8

— *My Thoughts* —

34

FACING A GIANT

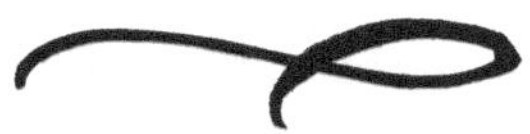

May 23, 2021. It was Sunday. Tired and depressed, I didn't do a lot—mostly cried and felt fearful. What a rollercoaster! I talked about faith and hope—and yet I was so afraid. Fear comes from Satan. I knew the drugs I was taking were affecting my thinking process—and Satan was taking advantage of that by instilling fear.

One way I fought fear during this journey was by reading the Bible. God's Word gave me hope, strength, and peace. I applied Bible stories to my cancer healing journey. The Scriptures give many examples of God's power.

I was in a battle. A battle against the giant of cancer. When the shepherd David was a young man, he faced a giant—Goliath. You can read about it in 1 Samuel 17. No one in Israel's army was willing to face this overwhelming giant. Then along came young David. He knew he couldn't defeat the giant in his own strength, but he trusted God. Here's what he said to the giant:

"You come to me with sword, spear, and javelin, but I come to you in the name of the Lord of Heaven's Armies—the God of the armies of Israel, whom you have defied. Today the Lord will conquer you, and I will kill you and cut off your head. And then I will give the dead bodies of your men to the birds and wild animals, and the whole world will know that there is a God in Israel!"

— 1 Samuel 17:45–46

David was small. He was not covered with armor. His weapon was a slingshot with five stones. But he was not trusting himself to meet this challenge—his trust was completely in God. And God won the battle.

This was another reminder that I was not facing the giant of cancer alone. The only answer was to trust God.

Be on guard. Stand firm in the faith. Be courageous. Be strong.

— 1 Corinthians 16:13

Reflections

Do you trust God? Have you taken your sickness to his feet for healing?

You may be facing the giant of cancer. Or the giant of loss or another kind of sickness. No matter what you are battling, the answer is the same. Concentrate on trusting God—and He will win the battle.

Spend time in God's Word. God gives so many examples of winning the battle for those who trusted him. David. Joseph. Moses. Joshua. And on and on. Ask him to speak to you through the Bible. You are in a real battle and must find hope and peace every day for months, and maybe even years.

Think again about the story of David and Goliath. David defeated the giant because he recognized God's power and strength and love. And he trusted in God, not himself.

It may be hard to believe you will live through this terrible illness and the treatments that may bring pain, sickness, diarrhea, nausea, weakness, and more. Some side effects come and go during treatment, and some occur every day until months after all treatments are complete. Test after test. Multiple biopsies, injections, needles, IVs, blood tests, scans— and more.

All this can bring fear to you—as it did to me. But don't give in to the fear. Don't quit fighting the battle. Speak God's Word to overcome the fear and pain. He will help you. Speak his name and call on him. Refuse to allow Satan to steal your joy and your faith! *Get behind me, Satan, for I am going to be victorious! I will hold my banner high. God is fighting this giant, and he has defeated it!*

Lord, bring me peace each day from the fear of what could be.

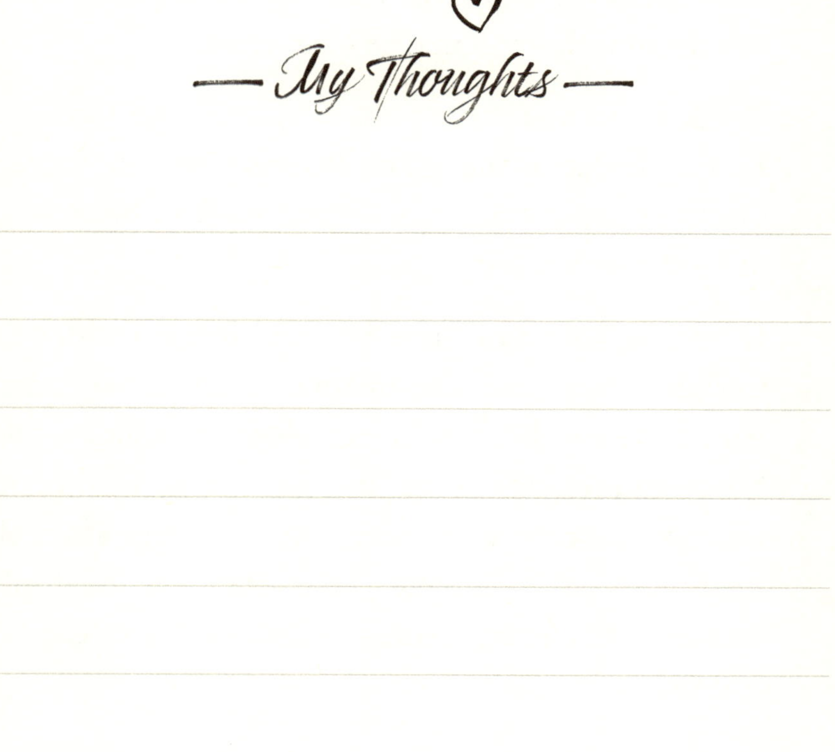

35

YOUR FEELINGS ARE NORMAL

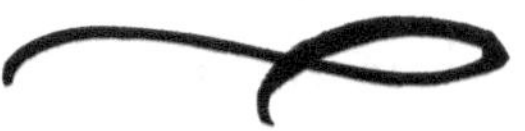

May 24, 2021. This was a better day, but in the middle of the night I had more diarrhea and became faint. When I was just lying down on the bathroom floor, David came to help with cool cloths. He helped me clean up and get back to bed. This was hard not only for me but also for my loving caregiver husband.

I tried to stay positive and help myself get around. The tears and fear came often. *Lord, please give me strength.*

> But each day the Lord pours his unfailing love upon me, and through each night I sing his songs, praying to God who gives me life.
>
> — PSALM 42:8

May 25. I was very tired and weak. This was the worst I'd ever felt in my life. In the evening, David and I went to the cancer support group, and they prayed over me. They were so encouraging and explained that cancer patients experience fear and a feeling of loss. The loss of what they could previously do, the loss of health, the fear of death. They experience sadness because of the changes in their lives.

May 26. That morning I broke out with shingles under my left arm, spreading around to my back. I sent pictures to the doctor, who confirmed it was shingles. She sent another prescription to the pharmacy. More medicine! I was overwhelmed with so many meds. I had a spreadsheet to keep track of what to take and when to take it. I was thankful that as a nurse I knew about many of the medicines and how to space them out for the most benefit.

May 27. Still very tired and weak, I slept two and a half hours in the afternoon. I had been napping each afternoon, but this was longer than usual. I was still experiencing rashes, a metal taste, lack of appetite, and nausea. Turning to God's Word, I meditated on Psalm 23. Verse 4 stood out.

> Even when I walk through the darkest valley, *I will not be afraid,* for you are close beside me. Your rod and your staff protect and comfort me. (Emphasis mine.)

"I will not be afraid." *But, Lord, I am afraid. So afraid. I need your help and strength.*

Reflections

Sadness and depression often oppress people in treatment for cancer. Some doctors in my hometown wanted me to take antidepression drugs, sleeping meds, and other medicines to help. But at MD Anderson, all the doctors encouraged me to be strong in faith and to talk about my feelings. They advised me to have faith and possibly get some counseling for depression. I attended a support group at one of the hospitals that helped me understand that everyone in treatment has fears. No one feels well, and every day is a battle. They had social groups where individuals shared about their journeys. I learned that every cancer journey is difficult. They also encouraged caregivers by holding dinners for them.

This group helped me realize the feelings I was having were normal. I heard others sharing their struggles. This gave me hope and calmed my fears. I was able to press forward without any antidepression meds. However, if you do need some medicines to help you get through this illness, please seek your doctor's help. There is no shame in taking that route. Everyone deals with the emotional side of the illness differently.

Know that what you are feeling is normal. I highly recommend you try to find a support group in your area. Ask your medical team about any they recommend.

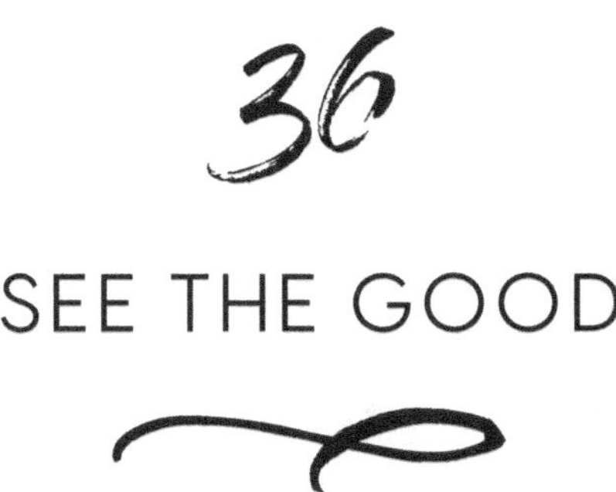

SEE THE GOOD

May 30, 2021. It was Sunday, and we went to church. During the service I was reminded that God is in control, and I was lifted up with peace. He has the final say in what happens. *Lord, please give me health the rest of my days on earth. I do not like sickness and pain. I would like to see my six grandchildren grow into young adults and graduate from school. I would love to watch their faith in Jesus grow. But, Lord, I am trusting your decision and I know your hand is on me.*

Our grandson Sawyer (five years old at that time) loved to sing "How Great Thou Art" to me. I recorded him singing it and added it as a ringtone on my phone.

God, you are speaking to me in many ways. First, there was the cross in our tree. Then came the double rainbow before my first chemo. And now our sweet grandson singing "How Great Thou Art."

I thought about the words. God's power is displayed in countless ways throughout our universe. He is greater than we can even imagine.

As Sawyer sings to me, I am reminded how great you are, Lord. Please hold me in your hand. Take away my fear. You know the days I have, and you have shown your power to me in the cross and rainbow.

May 31. Memorial Day. I still had some shingles on my left side. They were very painful, but I was thankful I had called the doctor right away so she could treat them to keep them from spreading. They were painful and burned and itched. I asked God over and over for peace, strength, and help.

Some of that help came from visiting with other cancer patients at a support group provided by another hospital. People there told me many things about their journeys— things I needed to hear and know. They reassured me my feelings were normal. What a blessing these groups were to both David and me.

I read a booklet a friend had sent. It reminded me God was there to help me.

"I am leaving you with a gift—peace of mind and heart. And the peace I give is a gift the world cannot give. So don't be troubled or afraid."

— JOHN 14:27

Reflections

Have you found a support group yet? I cannot begin to tell you how much it helped me to talk to other cancer patients. If you've not yet done so, I hope you will do that soon.

Also, remember to focus on the good things happening. Encouraging words here and there. People God sends to you at just the right time. Victories in the treatment procedures—even if they seem small. Each finished treatment that may bring terrible side effects but gets you closer to your goal.

And most of all, thank God for all these good things and for being with you. Even when you don't feel his presence, he is there. How can you know? Because he promised.

The faithful love of the Lord never ends! His mercies never cease. Great is his faithfulness; his mercies begin afresh each morning.

— LAMENTATIONS 3:22–23

My Thoughts

37

CAST YOUR CARES ON HIM

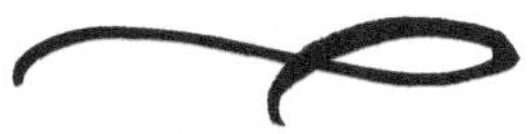

June 1, 2021. We had been in Texas for five weeks. David was leaving to go home and check on things. Because I was afraid of side effects and ending up in the hospital, I wasn't going to accompany him. I thought I was too weak, and I was worried about having diarrhea on the plane. However, at my sons' urging, at the last minute I decided to go. On the way to the airport, we bought some Depends in the event of diarrhea, and David arranged for wheelchair assistance at the airport. The staff was gracious and helpful.

When we arrived at our small home airport and they rolled me up to where my parents were waiting, I must have been quite a sight with no hair and wearing a head beanie. My face remained swollen, and the rash still covered my arms and face. Mom said, "Vicki, is that you?" (They didn't know I was coming with David and could hardly recognize me.)

"Yes, Mama, this is me. We will be home only a short time. We need to return for my second chemo in just a few days."

While at home, I took it easy and kept drinking my water. I so enjoyed getting to see some friends and family.

June 6. As we left the house to fly back to Texas, I cried and asked God to please let me come back home someday to enjoy family and our beautiful yard and home. I was still so afraid of the future.

When life sends us difficult times, we often feel as if others cannot understand what we're going through. But I knew many of my friends did understand and care. And I also realized others experience pain and suffering. Others have hurts and fears about the future. Others spend sleepless nights wondering what will happen. Others experience pain from relationships or physical or mental illness. Others have cancer.

I was especially reminded of this at a recent church service where many shared their needs—loss of jobs, marriages falling apart, suicide attempts, accidental deaths, serious illnesses. But I was also reminded of the healing power of Jesus. As the preacher knelt on the stage and held his hands up, praying for the needs, people all around the room joined him in prayer. The presence of the Holy Spirit was strong.

Reflections

If you are like me, in the midst of your suffering, you may lose sight of the fact that there are others around you in need. Recognizing those needs may make you feel a little less alone. The Holy Spirit may even draw you to whisper a prayer for them.

While on earth, we have bodies that get hurt. They get sick. They get breast cancer. But cancer is only one bad thing in life. Many other things—jobs, relationships, all kinds of illnesses, finances, and so much more—bring hurt and unexpected changes into our lives. Cancer means months and even years of treatment. It is a long journey with many ups and downs. Don't let this kill your faith! Believe God has a purpose, and he will get you to the other side. We must cast all our cares on him, for he cares for us. Stay strong!

Casting all your cares [all your anxieties, all your worries, and all your concerns, once and for all] on Him, for He cares about you [with deepest affection, and watches over you very carefully].

— 1 PETER 5:7 AMP

38

KEEP THANKING JESUS

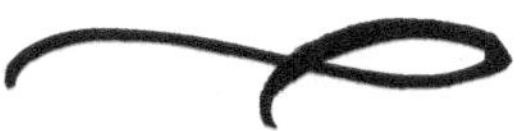

June 8, 2021. The night before my second chemo treatment, five-year-old grandson Sawyer had encouraged, "Nana, don't be afraid tomorrow for the doctor. It will not hurt! I have had a doctor give me a shot and it didn't hurt." All my grandchildren were so loving and encouraging. *Lord, please, may they each keep trusting you for my healing as they pray for me.*

My blood pressure was a little high before we left the house, so I took a pill to bring it down. Again, I had to enter the hospital alone because of COVID restrictions. They took everyone's temperature at the door and required masks and hand sanitizing. This day was so hot outside, I was concerned about David sitting in the car all those hours he would be waiting for me. Thankfully, he found some shade in the parking lot, where he sat, read, and prayed.

I felt alone and emotional as I went from the lab to the doctor's office to the infusion area. As I sat in the oncologist's office, the lab reports came over my phone. Praise the Lord—they all looked good! *God, you have blessed me with good lab results today. I am grateful and am asking for my body to be able to handle today's chemo without side effects that take me to the hospital.*

I was with the doctor about an hour. She thought I had done well after the first treatment—even with the side effects and trip to the ER! Feeling the tumor, she reported it had become softer, which meant it was responding to the chemo. I replied, "I am praying for it to be gone. God can do it."

"Yes, that has happened. God *can* do it!"

We then talked about faith and prayers from the nurses and doctors here at MD. Their encouragement uplifted me. My doctor said, "The power of the mind is very strong. Faith and positive thinking can heal the body."

Yes, God's Word tells us to hope and trust in him, no matter what things look like.

For we walk by faith, not by sight [living our lives in a manner consistent with our confident belief in God's promises].

— 2 Corinthians 5:7 AMP

I pray that God, the source of hope, will fill you completely with joy and peace because you trust in him. Then you will overflow with confident hope through the power of the Holy Spirit.

— Romans 15:13

Reflections

Open yourself to hope from heaven. Leaning on Jesus will help you face each day. Hope for healing … living … and feeling good again one day!

Keep your mind on Jesus. Thank him throughout this whole process—during the good and the bad. Thank him that the Holy Spirit is alive in you—directing, encouraging, and giving you strength to endure all you have to face.

God is our refuge and strength, always ready to help in times of trouble. So we will not fear when earthquakes come and the mountains crumble into the sea. Let the oceans roar and foam. Let the mountains tremble as the waters surge!

— Psalm 46:1–3

I used this powerful Scripture on cards I handed out with the prayer bracelets. You may want to do that with a Scripture you find yourself turning to often.

— *My Thoughts* —

39

SUFFERING PRODUCES FRUIT

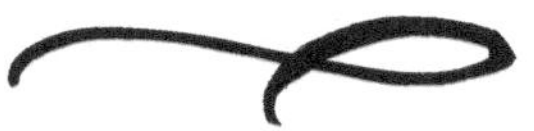

It was time for my second treatment. The routine would remain about the same for all six treatments before surgery, although some meds would be adjusted. First, the pre-meds. Part of this was through a subcutaneous injection given in my right thigh over six to eight minutes. It made my thigh very swollen for several days until it all absorbed.

This was followed by a chemo drug infusion that lasted from one to two hours. Then a saline flush of the port was followed by infusing the second chemo drug. Finally, another saline flush of the port.

After that, the OBI. Remember that from my first treatment? The wonderful Neulasta on-body injector on the left side of my abdomen? They alternated sides each time, so this time it was on my right side. Again, putting it in felt like a gunshot.

During the treatment, I was calmed by worship songs from my phone's playlist. I also responded to texts from people praying during the infusion.

By the time the procedure ended, I was so drugged out! They rolled me out in a wheelchair to David. Then off we went to Chick-fil-A for the chicken noodle soup that always tasted so good!

June 9. This time only my neck and face were red and hot to the touch. The doctor called in a prescription.

June 10. I had slept off and on. *Lord, thank you for any sleep. Please clear my mind and my fears.* A rash had developed on my feet, and I hurt all over. Even so, I walked a mile and a half at the Y and did some leg press exercises, followed by my usual two-hour afternoon nap. I had set a goal to give my body time to heal and to rest my mind every day. My mouth had begun to taste metallic, which made cold drinks taste terrible, but I drank seventy ounces of water each day. I finished the daily ninety-ounce requirement with a variety of choices.

Reflections

And we know that God causes everything to work together for the good of those who love God and are called according to his purpose for them.

— ROMANS 8:28

Really, God? I don't want to doubt your Word, but I can't find a way these things will bring good!

Do you ever feel like that? It's okay to ask questions. God knows how you are feeling anyway!

What is my purpose? What is God's purpose for this?

The Bible teaches that suffering produces fruit and silences the devil. It glorifies God. Makes us like Jesus. It helps us depend on God and refines our lives. It rebukes sin and enlarges our ministry.

We can rejoice, too, when we run into problems and trials, for we know that they help us develop endurance. And endurance develops strength of character, and character strengthens our confident hope of salvation. And this hope will not lead to disappointment. For we know how dearly God loves us, because he has given us the Holy Spirit to fill our hearts with his love.

— ROMANS 5:3–5

— My Thoughts —

40

WATCH FOR THE RAINBOW

June 11–20, 2021. The side effects continued. The rash on my feet peeled—it hurt to even take a shower. I had trouble sleeping and experienced times of being bone cold—even with six double-folded blankets covering me. I shook, my teeth chattered, and I hurt. (This coldness would be a repeating side effect until I finished my last treatment in 2022.)

June 12 was our fifty-first wedding anniversary. Chris and Amy took us out to dinner, but I was feeling too bad to really enjoy it. However, it gave me joy to reflect on the journey David and I had shared all those years—times of happiness, challenges, good times and bad—pressing on together as God planned. I was so grateful for a man who loves God and believes in his Word. His support and love encouraged me to look to the future when the treatments would be behind us.

Many times during this cancer journey, David sat through the night and read me Scriptures, played Christian music, or prayed over me. When I was too nervous or sad to read, he would hold my hand to enter God's presence and praise the Lord, who was walking with us.

On June 14, the diarrhea was so bad, I lay on the bathroom floor all night. David had to mop the floor, clean me up, and help me with my diaper. *Lord, this is so hard! Please give me strength and stop the diarrhea! Oh, Lord, please hear your servant's cry!*

As the days went on, the symptoms continued, and I had dizzy spells. I was on antibiotics, along with all the other meds, and felt drugged. I was still able to walk some at the Y or in the neighborhood. We were even able to take the grandkids to a waterpark—I sat inside and watched them. It brought me joy to see them have so much fun. Positive moments like that helped me stay focused on life. The love of a child can instill a desire to live—even when things look bleak.

The next several days, I continued feeling weak and tired, couldn't sleep, and still had some diarrhea. I was afraid my blood count would drop. *Lord. please hold on to me and give me strength to get through this!*

Reflections

So often as I struggled with the pain and sickness, I thought of Jesus and the agony he suffered for you and for me. I never came close to suffering the way he did—and he did it out of love. He knew the Father's plan. He asked for any way to avoid going through that but told the Father, "Nevertheless, not my will but yours be done."

I knew I needed to submit to God's plan. To his will. And trust him to help me through it. Again, those verses in Proverbs came to mind.

Trust in the Lord with all your heart; do not depend on your own understanding. Seek his will in all you do, and he will show you which path to take.

— Proverbs 3:5–6

We have a God we can trust in the midst of life's uncertainties. He brings up the sun and takes it down. He is in control of the moon and stars, rain and droughts. Even amid the treatments and horrible side effects and uncertainties, God was there holding my hand. And he is holding yours too. He is guiding your steps, giving you strength, giving you breath and life. Worship him! Give him thanks even when you don't feel thankful. Just as when he told Noah to build an ark on dry ground, God has purpose and perfect timing. Just wait and watch for the rainbow he will bring!

"Be still, and know that I am God!"

— Psalm 46:10

— *My Thoughts* —

41

HAVE SOME FUN!

June 21–26, 2021. It was the thirteenth day after my second treatment, and David and I set out for Galveston for "beach therapy." I wanted some quiet place where I could be alone to cry and sort out my feelings of fear and open my heart for God's direction and strength. Since I couldn't be in the sun, we walked along the beach in the cool of the morning or evening. And I enjoyed some reading time.

The side effects were still plaguing me, and my body smelled terrible! I had heard about the chemo smell, and now I was experiencing it, but I knew I must keep trying to live. And right now, that meant having a fun time with David. Along with walking on the beach, we enjoyed some sightseeing, ship watching, and shopping. We even did a round-shaped jigsaw puzzle together.

Day by day I trusted God to give me strength and peace of heart and mind. *Trust! God is in control.* I got stronger each day and was so thankful to be out walking.

God sent several people who blessed and encouraged me during this vacation. Some visitors. Some strangers in restaurants and on the beach. Many told me, "I will say a prayer for you" or "God will heal you—believe!" God is so good.

> I look up to the mountains—does my help come from there? My help comes from the Lord, who made heaven and earth! He will not let you stumble; the one who watches over you will not slumber. Indeed, he who watches over Israel never slumbers or sleeps. The Lord himself watches over you! The Lord stands beside you as your protective shade. The sun will not harm you by day, nor the moon at night. The Lord keeps you from all harm and watches over your life. The Lord keeps watch over you as you come and go, both now and forever.
>
> — PSALM 121

On June 26, we drove back to Chris and Amy's home. Along the way, we stopped at the MD Anderson hotel to get information about staying there during my September surgery.

Reflections

I encourage you to find a way to "get away from it all" for a few days. Have some fun! Your activities may be limited by your current health, but find some things you *can* do and enjoy. It will do you so much good.

I hope by now you have a circle of people praying for you. When you are up to it, be bold about providing specific issues for them to be praying about. You could do that in email or text or on CaringBridge. Or perhaps you have a prayer chain at church. Here is a list I did:

1) Pray against discouragement.
2) Pray for healing and tumor to be gone by third chemo treatment.
3) Pray for rest and peace!
4) Pray against side effects of rash, mouth sores, and diarrhea.
5) Pray for Chris's family as we live in their home long-term.
6) Pray for my parents at home, for strength and peace while I am away.
7) Pray for Shon's family, as they are in NC and long to be here to help.
8) Pray for David as he cares for me through the night and is having many arthritis problems.
9) Pray that God's power will be seen in healing and for my strength to endure through this process.

The earnest prayer of a righteous person has great power and produces wonderful results.

— James 5:16

42

PRAY THE SCRIPTURES

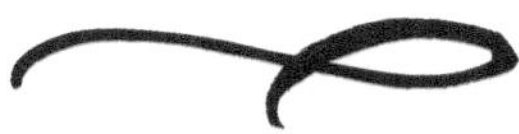

June 28, 2021. I was finally feeling stronger—and my head even felt clear! At the Y, I walked one and a half miles and did two weight machines. I could even taste my chicken sandwich and tea! I was so thankful, but I knew I needed to enjoy the moment. My third chemo treatment was scheduled for the next day. I thought of God's words to Joshua and knew they were for me at this moment.

> "This is my command—be strong and courageous! Do not be afraid or discouraged. For the Lord your God is with you wherever you go."
>
> — JOSHUA 1:9

June 29. Although I was not excited about having another treatment, I was so thankful that visitors could now come into the hospital, enabling David to be at my side for everything throughout the day! First, we took care of some scheduling and prescription business with part of the staff. Then we saw the doctor. She said I had done great and that the issues I'd had were normal—and even mild compared with many. *Really?*

She said if all went well, it would be okay for me to go home before the next treatment. I planned to find an oncologist at home in case of emergencies—also for radiation and any additional chemo needed after my surgery. (MD would oversee my treatments and medicines and do my follow-up tests for months and even years to come.) I quickly learned that many local doctors were not willing to work with MD Anderson patients, but I was finally able to get an appointment. In looking back, I was so thankful I had started with MD—I had been able to be diagnosed and start treatment so much more quickly than I would have been able to at home.

Back to that day's treatment. The same routine was followed. We spent seven hours at the hospital. David was blown away at how easily and efficiently we went from floor to floor, office to office, never waiting more than five minutes to be seen.

I mentioned earlier about the Bible cards and bracelets I handed out. On this day, I gave one of my regular nurses her third bracelet. She especially liked the prayer cards. She was always such a blessing to me—offering me Scriptures and Christian songs and praying for me. I hope you'll get a supply of Scripture prayer cards to hand out. You can make them or buy them at a Christian bookstore.

When the treatment was finished, we went back to the doctor's office to pick up an order for handicap parking. She explained I may get too weak to walk very far and probably would not have enough eyesight to drive. She just wanted to help me prepare for the possibilities.

Reflections

Treatment after treatment. Test after test. And the horrific side effects, with more to come. Do you sometimes cry and question why this is happening to you? I did. *What does God want me to learn? I can't see the end. How much more?* I counted down the treatments—the months, weeks, and days. Daily, I asked the Lord to make my blood work better, my diarrhea to stop, and the rashes to clear. I pleaded with him to keep my organs strong, to give me a clear mind, and to help my eyes see better and not water all day. One thing that encouraged me was to meditate on Scripture—and to pray it. That helped me focus more on Jesus and his love. That helped me choose to trust him and his plan, his timing. We've looked at Psalm 121 before. I encourage you to personalize it and pray it. Something like this . . .

Lord, as I look up, I am reminded that my help comes from you, the creator of heaven and earth. Lord, please don't let me stumble. I know you are watching over me—and you never sleep. Thank you for watching over me and standing beside me to protect me. Thank you for keeping me from all harm and watching over my life. Thank you for watching over me as I come and go—both now and forever.

— *My Thoughts* —

43

EVERY GOOD GIFT . . .

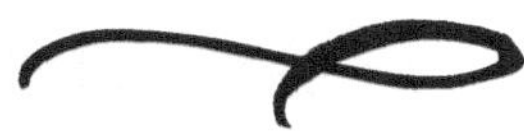

June 30, 2021. I did so well that day, we went shopping and I bought a new wig! I was so thankful for these times of relief from the side effects.

July 1. The OBI seemed to function well, but when it was empty, it began flashing red. None of the medical team understood why, so they decided to assume I had received the OBI medicine rather than risk giving me more. However, if I hadn't received enough, my white blood cell count could run low, lowering my immunity, so I would have to be very careful not to be exposed to any illness. Days ten to twenty following the treatment would be critical if the medication hadn't gone in properly. The doctor said we could still travel home as planned, but my local oncologist should monitor my blood counts. I actually felt good at this point.

July 2–19. After a good night's sleep, I packed for the flight home, and we headed for the airport. My foot was hurting because of a rash, but we made the trip without incident, and my parents were waiting at the airport when we landed. Fresh flowers and cards from friends awaited me at home.

During the two weeks at home, I often walked around the driveway to get exercise—and that seemed to help with the stress. Because of the chemo meds, my heart rate would go as high as 130 from just walking slowly for a few steps. Sitting helped it go back down. I did everything I could to protect my heart from chemo damage—resting, doing light exercise, eating right, drinking lots of water, and managing stress. I ate mainly celery with peanut butter, pretzels, oatmeal, bananas, and smoothies. Best of all, God's peace lifted me up and provided strength. Other side effects were similar to what I had previously experienced.

While home, I saw my new local oncologist to establish care for visits home and after my surgery. He was very kind and willing to work with MD in the months and years to come. The labs they did showed my count coming up—a happy surprise! That indicated the OBI must have given me my medicine!

David celebrated his seventieth birthday while we were home.

After seventeen days, we flew back to Texas. Our Houston kids had COVID, so we stayed at a motel.

Reflections

Although I would now be facing more tests and my fourth chemo treatment, this trip home gave me so much to be thankful for. Friends and family. Time to relax—and exercise in my own driveway! A kind doctor willing to work with MD. My blood count coming up.

I encourage you to take time to thank God for every good moment . . . or day . . . you have as you take this journey. You are probably finding, as I did, that some of the "little" joys can mean so much.

Here are two good Scripture passages to personalize and pray as you give thanks:

Whatever is good and perfect is a gift coming down to us from God our Father, who created all the lights in the heavens.

— JAMES 1:17

Your unfailing love is better than life itself; how I praise you! I will praise you as long as I live, lifting up my hands to you in prayer. You satisfy me more than the richest feast. I will praise you with songs of joy. I lie awake thinking of you, meditating on you through the night. Because you are my helper, I sing for joy in the shadow of your wings. I cling to you; your strong right hand holds me securely.

— Psalm 63:3–8

44

FOCUS ON THE SHEPHERD

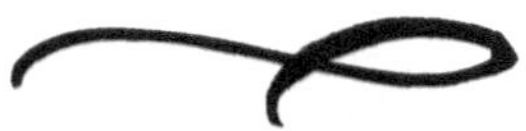

On our return to Texas, they did an ultrasound of my right breast to see how effective the first three chemo treatments had been. *Lord, please give me some encouragement in this report. May the tumor be gone or getting smaller!*

When we sat down with the doctor to discuss the results, she exclaimed, "Oh, my. Your test looks good!" The tumor had decreased 82 percent in size! And the affected lymph node was almost normal in size.

I praised the Lord for what he had done, and then we discussed the next treatments. I was halfway through the chemo treatments scheduled prior to surgery.

I praise you, Lord, for this good report. I believe you are removing the cancer!

I was trusting God that I could get through the next three chemo infusions with fewer reactions.

> Don't worry about anything; instead, pray about everything. Tell God what you need, and thank him for all he has done.
>
> — Philippians 4:6

July 20. Time for my fourth chemo treatment. I was so thankful David could be with me. My blood work was not within normal range, but the doctor said it was fine to proceed with the treatment. I had lost about ten pounds since treatment began. My potassium levels were low, so I needed a potassium IV.

Once again, I sat more than seven hours with IVs running. And, of course, they again packed my hands and feet in ice to help decrease nerve damage and neuropathy.

July 21. The usual side effects—and more—continued. The rash had spread to my arms and legs. My nails broke down in the quick and peeled. My fingers hurt so bad. On one foot I had no nails! No hair anywhere. And I was so bruised and sore from the previous day's injection. I was showering only about every three days because the water hurt so badly as it touched my body. I used a soft toothbrush and special paste that helped the sores in my mouth. My throat was tight and I had a raspy voice.

If we are thrown into the blazing furnace, the God whom we serve is able to save us. He will rescue us from your power, Your Majesty.

— DANIEL 3:17

God, I know you will protect me as I go through the fire with these tests and treatments. You will not let anything destroy me. I will walk through this fire and come out.

Reflections

Again and again, I pressed forward. Like a sheep, I went before God. I stood before the Shepherd, bowed my head, and allowed Jesus to do his work. When I focused on him, I chose to accept his leading and trust him. I knew he would bring me to a peaceful place of safety—and he will do that for you as well.

God is in control, and we must depend on him. Acknowledge you are weak and need God's strength. When fears about my health overwhelmed me, I filled my mind with God's love and goodness—and I prayed often.

For it is [not your strength, but it is] God who is effectively at work in you, both to will and to work [that is, strengthening, energizing, and creating in you the longing and the ability to fulfill your purpose] for His good pleasure.

— PHILIPPIANS 2:13 AMP

My Thoughts

45

LIVE WITH HOPE!

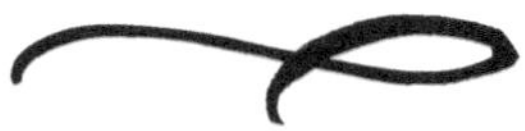

July 22, 2021. Flying home was an adventure. As I went through security, my bottom lit up! They quickly pulled me aside to say they would have to take me to the bathroom and check me over.

"No way! You can see I am sick and have no hair. I am a cancer patient in a wheelchair! I sometimes have uncontrollable diarrhea, so I am wearing Depends!"

"Okay."

This happened every time I wore Depends for our flight. I wondered why they didn't alarm for a baby or for the Depends in my suitcase! Why only when I was wearing them?

I was so thankful to be home in our quiet, small town. Since COVID was still in the area, we stayed rather isolated. I longed for the day we could return to church services and events we loved to attend.

I was blessed by many friends lifting me up daily in prayer, but I still feared the chemo treatments that lay ahead. I feared surgery, radiation, and more chemo after the surgery. I was afraid of reactions, more sickness, and even death. I longed for more hope.

Hope became my daily word. Hope! Hope that God would bless me through this journey and restore my health. Romans 15:13 meant so much to me—I have personalized the Amplified version here.

Lord, fill me will all joy and peace and help my faith to grow so that by the power of the Holy Spirit, I will abound in hope and overflow with confidence in your promises.

July 27. I saw my local oncologist. Among other things, we discussed the upcoming surgery. He thought I may be able to have a lumpectomy rather than a mastectomy. I felt we needed to wait and see what would happen with the next chemo treatments and the results of the ultrasound done before surgery.

One evening while we were home, my parents came for dinner. Dad said, "Sis, let's go for a ride!" We had been taking daily rides around the countryside to get me out and help me refocus on living. The world outside was so uplifting to me. The sky and grass helped me see God around me!

This time as we climbed into the car, Dad surprised me by saying, "Sis, you drive." I protested that I didn't think I could see well enough, but he encouraged, "You can do it!"

"Well, I guess I'm not dead yet, so I must do what I can to live."

I found my vision was fine for driving, and I began feeling alive! I started to believe I was getting better. I was so grateful for Dad's encouragement.

Reflections

I am certainly not encouraging you to do anything unsafe or against your doctor's instructions. However, I *am* encouraging you not to allow fear or a sense of helplessness to keep you from doing positive things you *can* do.

Think about your daily life. Have you allowed unnecessary boundaries to keep you from doing things you enjoy? If so, I hope right now you will pick one of those things and make immediate plans to get back into it. As time goes on, you may want to add others.

"For I hold you by your right hand—I, the Lord your God. And I say to you, 'Don't be afraid. I am here to help you.'"

— ISAIAH 41:13

My Thoughts

46

CHILDLIKE FAITH

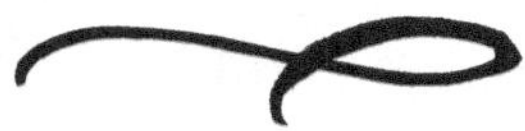

August 8, 2021. We flew back to Texas to prepare for the fifth chemo treatment. The time at home had been good for me. So often I could feel God filling me with hope, joy, and peace. The chemo drugs had inflicted my mind with confusion and fear, as they do to so many people, but during this time at home, my mind became clearer, and I felt stronger.

Some days I asked God the *why* questions. What had I done to have to go through this? Why me? My mom, in her usual sweet way, helped me. "This is life. None of us know what we will go through before we die. Everyone has a time to die, and life is not easy. We just have to believe and press on."

When we arrived in Houston, Chris and Amy were on a family vacation, so we were alone in their home. It was peaceful—but rather boring without the children!

The Bible talks about being like little children. What does that mean to us? I thought about trust and how our grandchildren trusted that Nana and Papa would love them, care for them, and spend time with them. Is that what it means to be like a child with God? Trust? Love? Spending time together?

I had always thought I trusted God, but in the midst of this difficult sickness, I wondered some days how much I was trusting. I thought about how excited our grandkids always were to see us. Did I get that excited about spending time with God? I knew I needed to build a closer relationship with him. I needed to trust him, to believe in his reliability, his truth, his strength, and his desire to care for me. I needed to show my love for him by spending more time with him, meditating on his Word, and talking to him.

> Then he said, "I tell you the truth, unless you turn from your sins and become like little children, you will never get into the Kingdom of Heaven."
>
> — MATTHEW 18:3

We can know God and believe in him. However, when we are struggling with illness and pain, it is hard not to ask why. I knew Satan was tempting me to feel sad and fearful and question God's love and faithfulness.

Lord, help me come to you with childlike faith. I believe, but please help my unbelief.

Reflections

Has your relationship with God changed during your illness? Maybe you have grown closer. Or perhaps you too have had some struggles with your faith.

God is the only one who truly understands what you are going through. He is the only one who knows what the future holds. His ways are not our ways, but his ways *are* the best ways. Only he can weave our struggles and victories during our life on earth into something that brings good. And only he loves us with truly unconditional love.

Can anything ever separate us from Christ's love? Does it mean he no longer loves us if we have trouble or calamity, or are persecuted, or hungry, or destitute, or in danger, or threatened with death? (As the Scriptures say, "For your sake we are killed every day; we are being slaughtered like sheep.") No, despite all these things, overwhelming victory is ours through Christ, who loved us. And I am convinced that nothing can ever separate us from God's love. Neither death nor life, neither angels nor demons, neither our fears for today nor our worries about tomorrow—not even the powers of hell can separate us from God's love. No power in the sky above or in the earth below—indeed, nothing in all creation will ever be able to separate us from the love of God that is revealed in Christ Jesus our Lord.

— Romans 8:35–39

Lord, help me trust you, your plan, and your timing. I know you love me and will never leave me. Help me know you better and trust you completely, no matter what.

— My Thoughts —

47

YOU HAVE A CHOICE

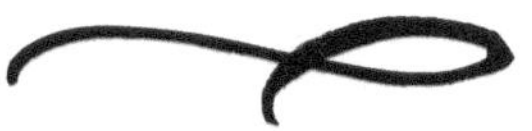

August 9, 2021. During my visits to my MD doctor, I was always excited to see my prayer cards hanging on her office wall. On this particular day, many of the staff told me they loved their bracelets and were reminded by them to pray for me. It was also a joy to give bracelets to other patients in the waiting room. (By the end of my final treatment, I had given away more than four hundred!)

On that day, my surgeon told me she was planning to place reflector markers in both breasts that week. They would light up under X-ray to reveal where the tumor was so they could determine if it was gone when it was time to prepare for surgery. They actually lit up under ultraviolet light and reflected out of my breast.

The doctor said if the tumor and the lymph node cancer continued to shrink, she thought she may be able to do a lumpectomy around the end of September. What great news! They also wanted me to get a COVID shot before the surgery.

CTs were done to see if my body had any cancer anywhere else—they were especially concerned about the liver. Praise the Lord! No new signs of cancer anywhere! They made some adjustments in meds and gave me another potassium IV.

I had more tests the next couple of days. My blood count was in a normal range—almost unheard of during chemotherapy. Heart tests showed my heart was strong. My weight was holding—I had lost no more than one or two pounds each treatment.

David and I rejoiced at the wonderful reports! God was at work!

> Everything he does reveals his glory and majesty. His righteousness never fails. He causes us to remember his wonderful works. How gracious and merciful is our Lord!
>
> — Psalm 111:3–4

Reflections

Each of us has thoughts or situations that bring us fear. We have a choice. We can choose to dwell on the fear and the what-ifs . . . or we can dwell on the good reports and, even more important, on God's love. I encourage you to think positive thoughts—cast out the fearful ones.

Your biggest enemy during this battle is fear, fear that leads to a sense of hopelessness.

Hope is a golden cord connecting us to heaven. During my cancer journey, this cord helped hold my head up, even on those days I felt the worst or received a discouraging report. Place your hope in Jesus. His love surrounds you. He is breathing his peace on you. Jesus is your hope.

And so, Lord, where do I put my hope? My only hope is in you.

— Psalm 39:7

May the God of hope fill you with all joy and peace in believing [through the experience of your faith] that by the power of the Holy Spirit you will abound in hope and overflow with confidence in His promises.

— Romans 15:13 AMP

48

THIS LITTLE LIGHT OF MINE

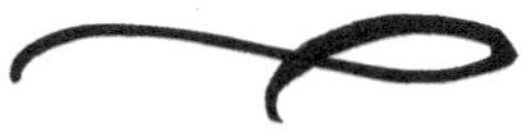

August 10, 2021. I received my fifth chemo treatment. It was the usual long process—and then David and I were off to Chick-fil-A for soup.

August 11. An MRI was done to place the reflectors in the node area and both breasts (my right breast because of the tumor and my left breast because of the calcification they would remove during surgery). The procedure was oh-so-painful. My breasts, sore from the various tests and treatments, had been bruised, iced down, and bound down with ace wraps. Once again, they were iced and bound with an ace wrap. I had to keep ice packs on them for forty-eight hours.

By the way, the first time we flew home after they were in place, they lit up going through security! I explained they were little lights to show where God was removing my cancer. So now both my boobs and my Depends were setting off alarms!

At this point I couldn't lie on my sides because my right breast was so sore and the left side was sore from the infusion port. The tube from the port went up my neck and down into my heart. It hurt to turn my head to either side, so I just limited my movement. And the days I had the OBI, I had to sleep only on my back. Before all this, I had loved sleeping on my left side, but at this point, I struggled every night to get comfortable. I looked forward to the day when all the treatments and surgery would be behind me and I could get comfortable again!

I kept praying for God to touch every spot and remove it completely. However, I knew he may choose to do that through the surgery rather than a miracle before then. *Lord, I know I must trust your decision!*

With this procedure done, my breasts would light up under ultraviolet rays. This seemed so funny to me! And then I thought about how God wants me to let the light of Jesus shine—all the time. I was reminded of a song I sang as a child: "This Little Light of Mine." Here are some of the verses I remember singing.

This little light of mine, I'm going to let it shine.
This little light of mine,
I'm going to let it shine, let it shine, let it shine.
Let it shine till Jesus comes,

I'm going to let it shine,
Let it shine, let it shine, let it shine.
Won't let Satan blow it out.
I'm going to let it shine, let it shine, let it shine.

Reflections

I believed it was fine to allow friends and loved ones to see my struggle with pain and fear. But I also wanted them to see that through the long struggle, I always strived to turn to Jesus and trust him. I wanted people to see his light still shining through me, no matter what. I wanted them to see his light encourage me, and strengthen me, and help me. And I wanted them to know he would do the same for them, no matter what they were going through.

Don't feel as if you have to hide the pain and fear from others. Only as they see that will they know how to pray for you. But also ask God to let his light shine through you to encourage others and bring them hope.

I pray reading about my journey will bring you hope! That you will look around you for God's blessings and signs of his love, protection, and hope. And that even through your journey, his light in you will shine.

"You are the light of the world—like a city on a hilltop that cannot be hidden. No one lights a lamp and then puts it under a basket. Instead, a lamp is placed on a stand, where it gives light to everyone in the house."

— MATTHEW 5:14–15

— *My Thoughts* —

49

FOCUS ON TODAY—
AND ON JESUS

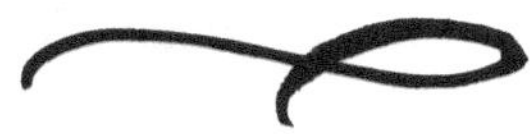

August 12, 2021. I had the COVID shot required for surgery. In a few days we would fly home and then return to Texas on August 28.

During the time at home, I was even more tired than usual with the combination of the chemo treatment and COVID shot. And I hurt all over. My mind was cloudy. Thinking ahead, I knew it may take up to a year for all the side effects to go away.

I felt overwhelmed with what I'd already gone through and fearing what would happen next. *Lord, only you can open the way and do a miracle for me. I lie at the foot of your cross and ask for healing.*

Then I began to reflect on how much David and I had to be thankful for. God had held us up through dark, sleepless nights with Scripture and songs. I had Christian doctors who encouraged spiritual peace. And so many friends who texted, sent cards, called, dropped off food, and—most important—prayed. A place to stay at our son's during treatment. And so, so much more.

August 28. We flew back to Texas. I was still weak, sick, and nauseous and had lots of diarrhea. Although I continued to cry at times, I was handling things somewhat better. But the struggles were still there. *What if I go through all this and then still die?* After all, I knew I would die someday. Everyone does. *Lord, I am just so thankful you are in charge.*

I couldn't imagine not getting to live to see my grandchildren grow, but I knew I was not alone—many face such fears. I was thankful for the two support groups where we shared our fears and anxieties and suffering and learned all those feelings were normal! I was able to tear away from my focus on fear and worry and concentrate on Jesus when I thought about what he said about worry.

> "And who of you by worrying can add one hour to [the length of] his life?"
>
> — MATTHEW 6:27 AMP

Reflections

Do you sometimes feel as if you are the only one in the world going through such physical and emotional trauma? Do you think you must be handling things poorly because you are experiencing fear and doubt?

I am here to tell you, all this is normal for people walking a journey with cancer. You are certainly not the only one. If you've not yet found a cancer support group, I urge you to look for one today. Check with your church, your medical team, or a local cancer organization. I can't begin to tell you how much the groups helped me. I was with people who were living it—so we all understood one another.

Like me, you may be experiencing fear and dread of dying. The thought of leaving loved ones behind can be devastating. But if you have received Jesus as your Lord and Savior, when you do die, you will simply be stepping into his arms and living in a place so incredible you can't even begin to fathom how wonderful it will be.

I am certainly not saying to give up. Jesus is the healer! And he may have more for you to do on this earth. Pray for healing. Ask others to pray for your healing. But be willing to pray, as Jesus did, "Not my will but yours."

And then begin to take one day at a time. Remember what Jesus said.

"So don't worry about tomorrow, for tomorrow will bring its own worries. Today's trouble is enough for today."

— Matthew 6:34

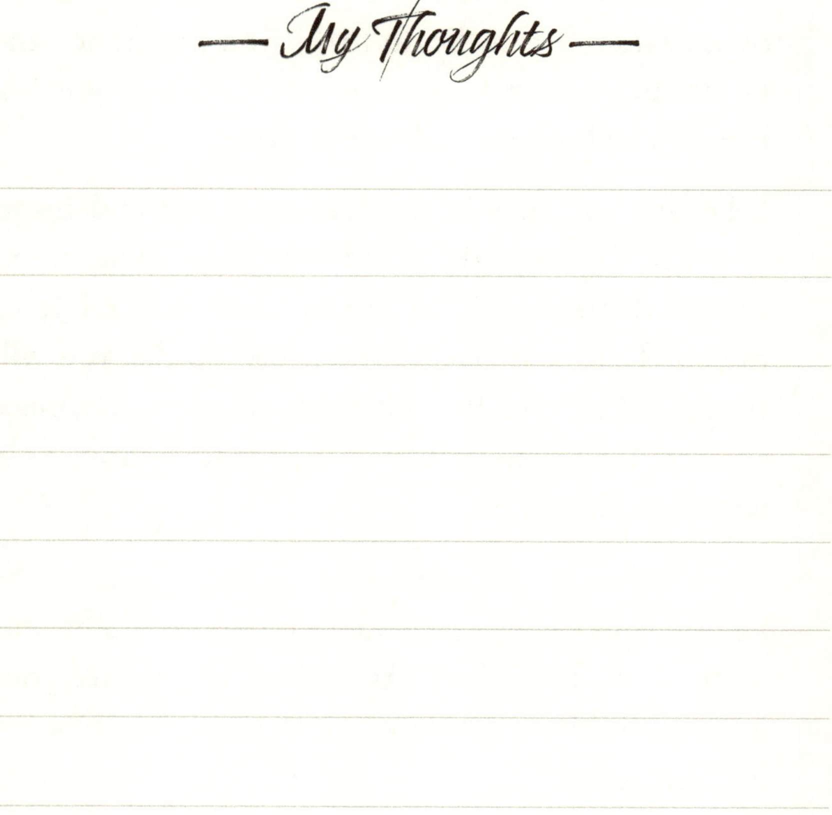

50

FINAL TREATMENT BEFORE SURGERY!

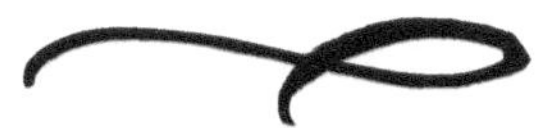

August 30, 2021. The day had finally arrived! The final infusion before surgery. The last of the four Red Devil drugs.

Since I planned on having my next fourteen rounds of chemo at home over the next year, I would not be seeing these nurses again. Although I had already shared prayer cards and bracelets with them, I wanted to do something else to express my appreciation for all their support, love, and prayers, so David and I arranged to provide deli sandwiches, brownies, and chips for all the staff in the infusion area. Chris helped by picking it all up and delivering it.

The routine was the same as the previous five treatments, but the OBI seemed to hurt more than usual when they put it in my abdomen. I was so grateful to God that this would be the last time for those ice packs on my feet and hands.

After the infusion, I celebrated by ringing the cancer bell! Many of the nurses came to cheer me on. It was a good day, but I felt terrible. *This isn't the end. I still have so much more to go!*

David teared up as I rang the bell—he was so happy for me! I was thankful for his encouragement and care along the way. Although he was celebrating with me, I knew he was tired and, like me, wondering what lay ahead.

Since this round of chemo had come to an end, after my second COVID shot, we flew home for about two weeks. Then we would return for tests and preparation for surgery, scheduled for September 30.

When we got home, I was super weak and experienced the usual side effects. As always, David took such good care of me. He worked hard to keep me eating and drinking. Along with all the physical care, his encouragement and efforts to keep me calm when I became upset or fearful or cried uncontrollably with fear meant so much to me.

As I gained more strength at home, one day I told David, "I am not dead yet, so I am going for a ride! I will be back later." After climbing into my '66 Mustang I'd had since

I was sixteen, I pulled out of the driveway. And I felt alive! It was wonderful! I picked up a friend. We bought sandwiches and picnicked at a beautiful park, where we enjoyed a good visit. I was so refreshed within my spirit!

Another bright spot during this time was an early seventieth birthday celebration (my birthday would be a few days before surgery). Because of COVID and my need to be well for the surgery, a dear friend planned a "drive-by" seventieth birthday wish in our driveway! What a blessing!

Reflections

During a cancer journey, both the patient and the caregiver face many struggles. I encourage both you and whoever is helping you to meditate on these two Scriptures often. They are really hard to obey when you are in a health battle—but so important.

"This is my command—be strong and courageous! Do not be afraid or discouraged. For the Lord your God is with you wherever you go."

— JOSHUA 1:9

Be kind to each other, tenderhearted, forgiving one another, just as God through Christ has forgiven you.

— EPHESIANS 4:32

Another reminder—when you can, do something fun! Getting out . . . driving my Mustang . . . picnicking with a friend. That did me more good at that point than any medicine could have. Remember to be kind, not only to others, but also to yourself!

51

TALKING TO GOD

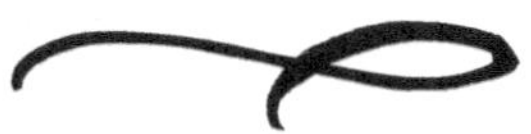

As I was preparing both physically and emotionally for surgery, I thought about the previous months. Five months had passed since I had been diagnosed with breast cancer. It had been a hard journey, but God had been with me through every chemo treatment and had held my hand day and night. And I knew he still was. He had shown his love and power throughout the trial, and I knew he would continue to do that throughout surgery and the remaining treatments.

I longed for days of health and a happy heart every day. I determined to press on with his strength and his power over heaven and earth. I would continue praying for healing.

Here was my prayer that day . . .

Lord, I ask you to give me normal blood work, a calm mind, and no depression. Lord, pull me through with positive thoughts and sleep at night that is peaceful.

Lord, may you speak your healing power over me today. I pray to be happy and positive.

Lord, may my blood count come up and my organs stay strong. Cause the rash all over my body to decrease. Lord, may I have less diarrhea and no bleeding of organs, a clear mind, and less crying and confusion with less depression. May my nails not peel or break off. I pray I can manage the pain and reactions with fewer drugs. Help me begin eating better with less metal taste in my mouth. Please remove all the mouth sores. Lord, you know this is not my complete list of reactions, but these are the ones that have troubled me every day for all these months. Lord, make my body strong for surgery and prepare it for the next rounds of chemo and radiation. I am leaning on you, Lord.

Lord, I long to share more anniversaries with David and see all our grandchildren graduate from high school. Lord, I want to be available to help my parents as they continue to age. I ask you to help me be a light of encouragement to other cancer patients. I long to live for your purpose.

Lord, I pray to leave a legacy of faith for my family. Give me health and healing from this cancer. May I be able to go through this illness! Lord, protect all my organs from any damage from the treatments. I love your power and your promises of eternal life when I leave this earth.

Reflections

I encourage you to press on through the pain, weakness, and fear. Someday it will be finished. We must trust his plan and his timing for our journeys. Christ is the victor. God never loses. He is powerful and is in control. He is not defeated. Jesus is on the throne over all!

Therefore we do not lose heart. Though outwardly we are wasting away, yet inwardly we are being renewed day by day. For our light and momentary troubles are achieving for us an eternal glory that far outweighs them all. So we fix our eyes not on what is seen, but on what is unseen, since what is seen is temporary, but what is unseen is eternal.

— 2 Corinthians 4:16–18 NIV

Sometimes you may not feel his presence or his love, but your feelings don't always discern truth. God's Word is truth. Read his words. Say his words aloud. Keep Satan away with God's Word. Meditate on his words. Pray his words.

God wants you to talk to him—and listen. Even when you don't feel like it, keep that channel of communication open. Just talk to him. Sometimes you may even find it helpful to write your prayers. I encourage you to do that right now. Let him know how you feel. Tell him your fears and desires. Ask him to help you have faith to trust his plan and his timing. Thank him for being with you. Pick up a pen and write to him right now!

— *My Thoughts* —

52

LOOK FEAR IN THE FACE

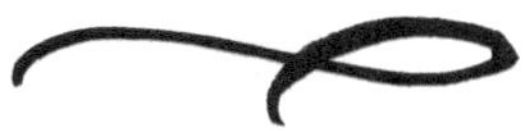

September 19–20, 2021. We flew back to Houston on September 19, and I began the pre-op tests the next day. This week I would find the answer to many of my questions about what was to come. I would have a full body MRI; chest X-rays; a mammogram, MRI, and ultrasound of both breasts; an EKG and ECHO of my heart; a COVID test; and many blood tests.

That first day began with blood work. Praise the Lord! My blood count was about the same as the previous time. I wouldn't need an IV or blood before surgery!

The nurse for those tests was one I'd had before and gifted with a bracelet. She greeted me with a hug, saying, "I wear my bracelet often and remember to pray for you. Today I have something for *you!*" She handed me a lovely daily devotional book with a special message from her written inside. That became a steadfast daily devotion for me during all the months that followed. I recorded daily happenings in each devotional.

Next, I went to the infusion area to get the first of my next fourteen rounds of chemo shots in my thigh. I received only two of the four drugs that had been given in the first six treatments—but I knew these two drugs had caused many of the side effects. Again, my blood work had revealed low potassium, so I had a potassium IV.

September 21. This was the day for the mammogram, ultrasound, MRI, and chest X-ray. These tests put a lot of radiation in my body—more than a person should be exposed to in a year! But sometimes we have to do things like that when we are sick.

The mammogram was done at eight o'clock—they took a lot of pictures. The tech had assisted me with my previous mammograms and biopsies and had received one of my bracelets. She told me, "I wear your bracelet and never forget to pray for you." I gave her another one. At the end, the radiology doctor joined us. "This is good news. The doctor will explain it to you later." Praise God! Encouraging words!

Next came the MRI and chest X-rays. I hadn't met these techs before. They were running behind, rushing in and out, so I hadn't found a chance to give them bracelets. Then another tech (one I knew) saw me. "Hi, Mrs. Earhart. I wear my bracelet every Sunday to church and say a special prayer for you. You remember God's already taken care of this, and you are healed!" I handed her bracelets to give the two new girls. We parted with a hug.

Reflections

If you are not already doing so, I hope you will begin giving out bracelets and prayer cards. The recipients are blessed—and many of them, if not all, will be reminded to pray for you.

At this point, so much unknown loomed ahead. What kind of surgery would I have? Would the radiation cause as many problems as chemo had? And what would the outcome be?

You are probably asking a lot of questions too. It's only natural. When worry and fear began to overtake me, I made every effort to refocus on thoughts and Scriptures like these:

Can worrying add an hour to my life? Why do I worry? God has a plan. I will rest in his hands, and he will hold me. You, Lord, know the days I have. I must be joyful for each day I have.

"I am leaving you with a gift—peace of mind and heart. And the peace I give is a gift the world cannot give. So don't be troubled or afraid."

— JOHN 14:27

Stay strong. Let go of things I cannot change. My experience will be a beautiful gift of hope. God is in control! Don't take my eyes off him! I will look fear in the face—I will live through this horror! I must do the thing I think I cannot do!

God's power goes before me!

> Never lagging behind in diligence; aglow in the Spirit, enthusiastically serving the Lord; constantly rejoicing in hope [because of our confidence in Christ], steadfast and patient in distress, devoted to prayer [continually seeking wisdom, guidance, and strength].
>
> — Romans 12:11–12 AMP

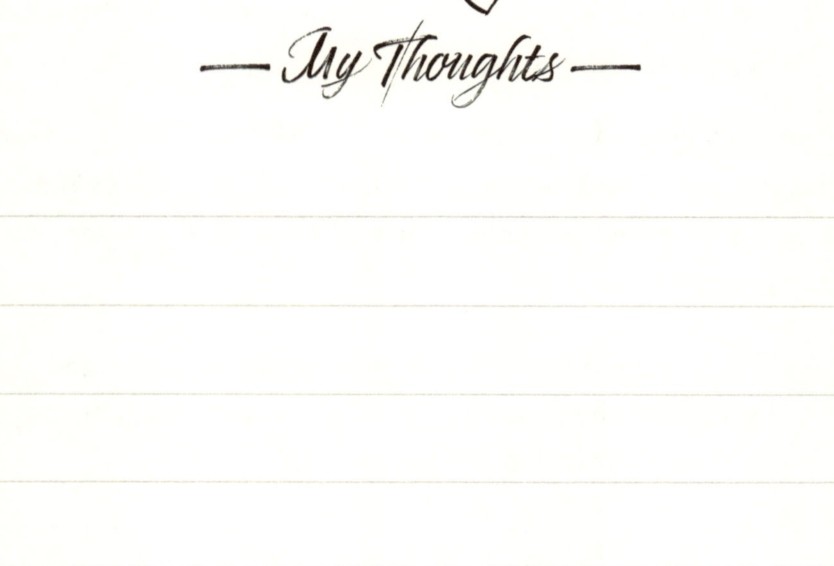

53

MASTECTOMY

September 22, 2021. This was my final appointment with my surgeon before the actual surgery. She greeted us as she came into the room. "The good news is the cancer is all gone. You had great results from the chemo! So great that the large tumor in your right breast is dead and basically gone. However, it has left small salt-size dead cancer in the breast."

Because there were multiple small dead pieces, she did not think it wise to try to do a lumpectomy. Since my breast was small, she believed that to get all the small pieces and good margins around the area would take more than half the breast. Not only would it be difficult to be sure they got all the cancer, but that kind of surgery would leave me with a misshaped breast.

Another argument against doing only a lumpectomy was that the breast still had several milk glands with calcification in them—another gland like that had led to the cancer to begin with. When the pickleball had hit a gland, cancer was already growing in it. It broke open, giving more room for the cancer to grow. There were still other glands with calcification in them, and chemo doesn't kill anything inside a milk gland.

We discussed doing a right mastectomy, and I began to cry. I was so upset—I was not prepared for the decision. She said she'd leave us alone to decide how to proceed.

There was no cancer in the breast. God had answered that prayer. But why a mastectomy?

I was so sad, but then I began to focus on the fact that the cancerous tumor was gone. God had healed it! And he would continue to heal. I had to trust him with no reservations. This wasn't the plan I had in my mind, but he was in control. Apparently, this was part of his plan— and his plan is always best.

When the doctor returned, we told her we trusted her and would go ahead with the right mastectomy. She would also remove the milk glands in the left breast— they had calcification but no cancer.

We would not know for sure about the lymph nodes until the surgery was in process.

Reflections

When we are seeking God's help, it's so easy for us to try to "help." We figure out how he is going to fix things. Then when his plan doesn't match ours, we are really let down. Has that happened to you?

There are many Scriptures that remind us to trust his understanding and not our own.

Trust in the Lord with all your heart; do not depend on your own understanding. Seek his will in all you do, and he will show you which path to take.

— PROVERBS 3:5–6

"My thoughts are nothing like your thoughts," says the Lord. "And my ways are far beyond anything you could imagine. For just as the heavens are higher than the earth, so my ways are higher than your ways and my thoughts higher than your thoughts.

— ISAIAH 55:8–9

When something happens during your journey that is different from what you had envisioned, try not to see it as a setback. Remember that God is in control. His plan may look different than yours—but his plan is always best.

My Thoughts

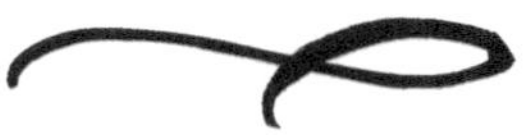

PREPARING FOR SURGERY

September 24, 2021. I had an EKG and ECHO. All was good! My heart was holding up strong.

The surgery was scheduled for September 30. I would spend one night in the hospital. Then David and I would spend two nights in the hotel at the hospital. After that, we planned to go to a beach house in Galveston for a week of healing. The length of our Texas stay would be determined by the recovery period after surgery.

September 26. I was blessed with a big happy birthday sign in my son's yard this morning! It was so beautiful and included words of encouragement: *Happy Birthday, Believe, 70th, Nana, Pray, Joy, Hope, Cure, Mama Is Queen.* It was also adorned with pictures: a cancer ribbon, butterflies, a birthday cake, and packages. What joy it brought!

September 27 was my actual birthday. The day began with more lab and COVID tests. Then I had lunch with Judy, after which we went shopping for a dress to wear to my niece Marylee's wedding in October. I was planning on getting home for that! I was blessed with many special birthday cards and gifts and thankful for so many blessings from family and friends. The next day David took me to lunch for yet another birthday celebration!

September 29. After going to lunch and shopping for shoes, David and I headed to the MD Anderson hotel in the main hospital building. It is in the heart of Houston, about ninety minutes from our son's home.

Although I was feeling better, the tears poured that day. I still had diarrhea and was weak. I had several things to do that night to prepare for surgery the next day, and David and I needed to go to bed early since we had to be at the admissions office by four o'clock the next morning.

After I had done all the showering, special scrubs, and other surgery preparations, David handed me a box full of get-well cards from friends and family. I was overwhelmed with all the wishes, prayers, and words of encouragement. Tears continued to flow again.

Reflections

I had definitely reached another emotional peak. There had been many of those during this cancer journey. I am sure you are experiencing that during your journey as well. *What will happen? Will there be complications? Will they get it all? How much pain and sickness will I have? Will I really get well—or am I approaching the end of my life on earth?*

In my prayer request list to my prayer warriors that week, I included this statement: "I shall press forward. God is the one with the plan. As much as I wish and pray for healing, it is his decision. As I say over and over, someone has to be in charge. God is the one who began this world and made life, so he is the power over each person's life."

I would live with hope. Hope for healing. But I would also trust God. *I believe with all my heart that God loves me and wants what is best for me. I believe his plan—even when I don't understand it—is the perfect plan. And I trust him.*

The Lord is a shelter for the oppressed, a refuge in times of trouble. Those who know your name trust in you, for you, O Lord, do not abandon those who search for you.

— Psalm 9:9–10

This I declare about the Lord: He alone is my refuge, my place of safety; he is my God, and I trust him.

— Psalm 91:2

— *My Thoughts* —

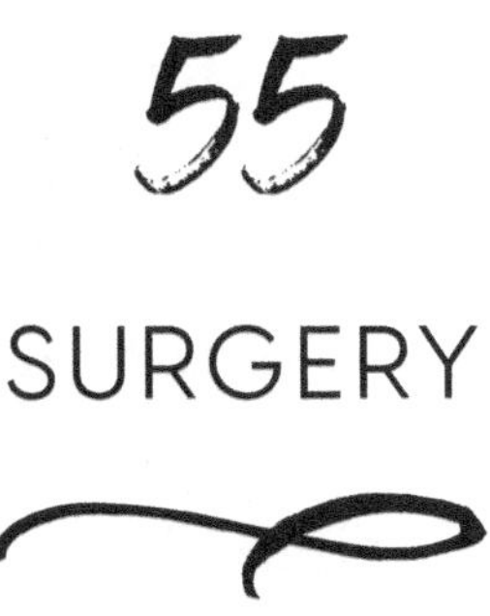

SURGERY

September 30, 2021. The long-awaited day had finally arrived. Surgery. David and I walked the long halls from the hotel to admissions at 4:00 a.m. After a few questions and paperwork, they took us to the pre-op area.

My doctor came in to visit and answer any questions we may have. I believed God had put me in good hands. David kissed me good-bye, and they rolled me to surgery at 6:50. We went down a long hallway, turning several corners, and then entered a large operating room. They had me move over to the operating table and put me on oxygen. Someone began the medicines in my IV—and I was fast asleep.

This was the official description of my surgery: Targeted axillary node dissection, excision biopsy of breast lesion on left breast, 2 mm calcification in left breast and milk glands, right segmental mastectomy with axillary lymph removals.

I was in surgery about four and a half hours and then in recovery. My doctor talked with David to update him and said they'd let him know when I went to a room. When there was still not a room available at 2:00 p.m., they let him come sit with me in recovery. I finally went to a room at 8:40 that night. After helping me settle in, David returned to our hotel room to get some much-needed sleep.

During surgery, the doctor was shocked to find two lymph nodes still with cancer. To get clear margins, she removed seventeen lymph nodes. More tests would be done on all the removed tissue, but the doctor reassured me that she had taken all the cancer out—the lab kept testing it during surgery until there was no more sign of cancer. Praise the Lord!

I would return to the doctor about October 13 for the drains to be removed and to get the final reports and learn details about future treatments. She said I would probably need to take the maximum radiation and another chemo drug every three weeks until July of 2022.

Reflections

Praise God! This had been a blessed day! The surgery was complete. The cancer was gone—and yet I somehow felt disappointed. I kept telling myself not to be sad. Not to be afraid. But so much still lay ahead—healing from surgery, radiation, and more chemo. I remembered that I must take one day at a time.

Do not be anxious or worried about anything, but in everything [every circumstance and situation] by prayer and petition with thanksgiving, continue to make your [specific] requests known to God. And the peace of God [that peace which reassures the heart, that peace] which transcends all understanding, [that peace which] stands guard over your hearts and your minds in Christ Jesus [is yours].

— PHILIPPIANS 4:6–7 AMP

I knew Satan was distracting me from the blessings I'd just experienced by implanting disappointment, worry, and fear.

Stay alert! Watch out for your great enemy, the devil. He prowls around like a roaring lion, looking for someone to devour.

— 1 PETER 5:8

And I determined all the more to resist the devil and keep my eyes on Jesus—my Savior, my healer, my God.

So humble yourselves before God. Resist the devil, and he will flee from you.

— JAMES 4:7

56

GOD HAS THE PLAN

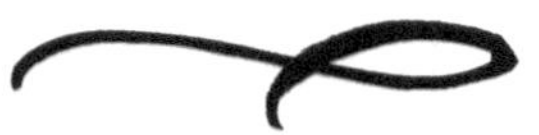

October 3, 2021. Three days had passed since surgery, and it was time to leave the hotel and head for our house rental on the beach in Galveston. First, we met Chris, Amy, and the children for lunch at a pizza place. From there, we set out on the drive.

We had a large house on the water with a wonderful view. Every day David and I read and sat on the deck. We took walks a couple of times each day and drove to the beach. Although I couldn't get into the water, we walked the sand area some.

I didn't have any pain but continued to take pain meds and a prescription, along with Tylenol or Ibuprofen. I was very tired and not eating well but able to move my arm. I still cried a lot and was fearful about the upcoming pathology report.

A few days later, the doctor's office called to tell me there was still some cancer in two of the lymph nodes, but the large tumor was dead. Since the lymph nodes had 5 percent cancer in one and 10 percent in the other, I would need some different chemo for the next fourteen rounds of treatment. I would also need the maximum amount of radiation—thirty rounds over six weeks, beginning six to eight weeks post-op.

I was overwhelmed! My mind and heart hurt. I had asked God to totally heal me. I was not being thankful for what God *had* done but focused on what I still had to go through. How could I be so ungrateful? I prayed repeatedly for peace and joy, not sadness, and spent a lot of time in my Bible.

Since I had faith in God, I couldn't believe the questions haunting me. *Why am I going through this? What did I do? Why can't I find peace? Why didn't God remove all the cancer?*

I knew God understood my disappointment, questions, and doubts. My days were now spent on the deck reading and praying—looking for answers. David encouraged me to be happy for all God had done already. Still, I struggled.

October 7. Mike, a young man who had lived with us while he attended Ozark Bible College in Joplin, came for a visit. When I told him I was heavyhearted, he reassured me that was normal for all I had been through. He said to hang on to my faith because my faith would heal me. We talked and shared more, and I felt more at peace by the time he left.

Reflections

During this time, I repeatedly told myself I must not fear. *I must trust God, have faith, and cast my cares on him. God is my strength. He will not let me be shaken. I must lean on him—his grace will hold me! I must have joy and hope by fixing my eyes on Jesus. Lord, bind Satan from me. Do not let him steal my joy. Give me strength.*

> I shed a multitude of tears and struggled through many prayers before I finally realized that God had the plan! He does not need medicine, doctors, or chemo to heal. Sometimes he works through those things, but he has the power to wipe out any sickness with a word. Sometimes he takes us down a valley to bring others blessings.
>
> Yes, I had thought the *doctor* would tell me the cancer was gone, but God wanted me to know *he* was saying it was gone! He had promised me he would be with me through the first rainbow back before any treatment had begun.

Do I believe? I must trust he has healed me. But wait . . . I must accept his plan, his way.

> Each of us must work at our faith. We must stand firm, for the devil is prowling around to see who he can devour.
>
> Put on all of God's armor so that you will be able to stand firm against all strategies of the devil.
>
> — EPHESIANS 6:11

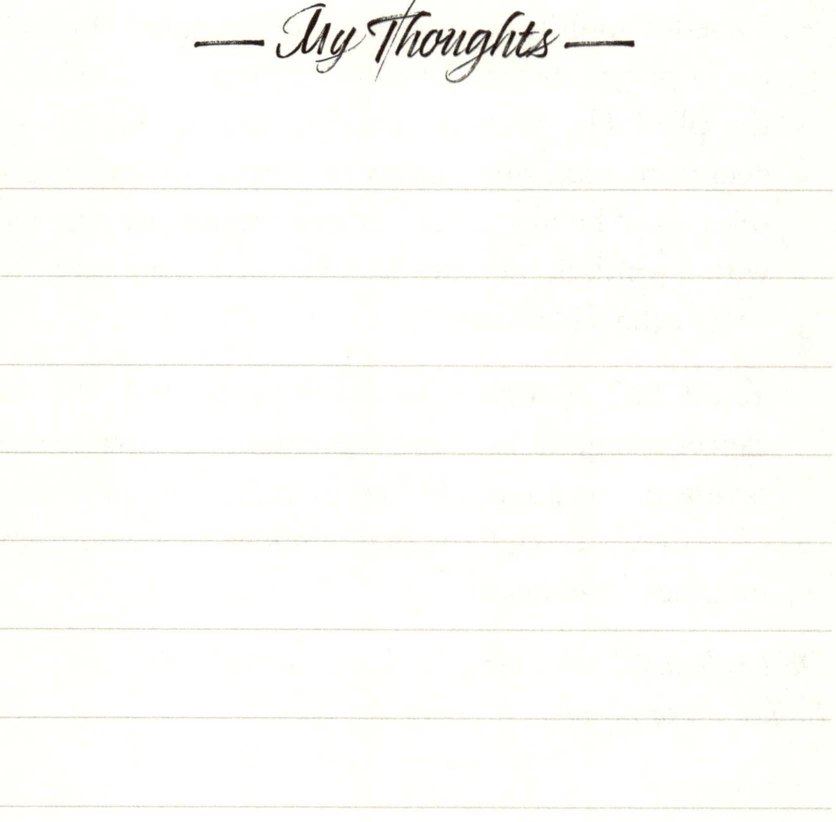

57

ONE HUNDRED PERCENT GOD!

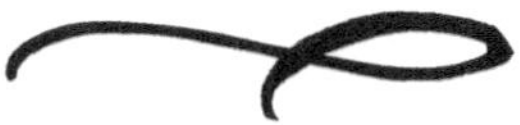

October 11, 2021. My first appointment that day was with my surgeon. She was able to remove one drain because of decreased drainage. She left the other drain in, but we would still be able to travel home, and my Joplin doctor would remove it when the surgeon gave the okay. I would stay in touch with her online (MyChart) or by phone.

October 12. I saw my oncologist, who talked to me about the cancer and what to expect. She said my cancer was stage 1B, grade 2. The various numbers indicated triple positive cancer and were middle of the scale for aggressive invasive ductal carcinoma.

Triple positive cancer can return in the lungs or liver. The next one to three years cancer-free would decrease the possibility of its return. By five years there would be almost no possibility. My doctor predicted a possible 5 percent chance of a return in my breast and 10 percent in another organ. Because of these low percentages, we would do body scans and other tests only if I showed any symptoms. I would take an anti-estrogen drug for five years—possibly up to ten years if studies continued showing benefits from longer use.

Next, I saw my heart doctor and learned all heart tests showed good results. I would be retested at home in about three months.

It was time to return home. We packed our things at Chris's home. David and I knew it would be hard leaving him and Amy and their kids after living there most of the time for six months! We were so grateful for all they had done. It was a tearful good-bye.

Reflections

As we received the doctors' reports, David reminded me how positive the numbers were that the cancer would *not* return. I wrote the positive numbers in my journal (see below) and continued to lift them up to God in praise. I also chose to leave everything in his healing hands. God would do as he planned—and his plan is always best.

For everything there is a season, a time for every activity under heaven. A time to be born and a time to die.

— Ecclesiastes 3:1–2

The doctor gave me the percentage possibilities of cancer returning. After David's encouragement, I changed those to percentages it would *not* return— and chose to dwell on that.

- 100 percent chance that God has this
- 95 percent chance of no return to left breast
- 95 percent chance of no return after radiation
- 97 percent chance of no return because of no family history
- 95 percent chance of no return to other organs since only two lymph nodes tested positive
- 95 percent chance of not going to other organs
- 90 percent chance of no spread to other parts of my body

Looking at the numbers this way gave me hope. Hope . . . because the 100 percent is God! There is no other fact that strong.

Do you have hope?

This hope is a strong and trustworthy anchor for our souls. It leads us through the curtain into God's inner sanctuary. Jesus has already gone in there for us.

— Hebrews 6:19–20

My Thoughts

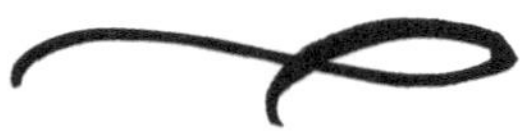

58

A DOUBLE RAINBOW

October 13–14, 2021. We took two days to drive home. I did well and was pain free for the trip. My mom and dad came to see us just as we arrived home. They brought sandwiches and helped us unpack. It was so good to see them. We found food in our refrigerator—brought by caring friends. One precious friend had even cleaned the house! We also discovered flowers and cards welcoming us home.

As my parents were pulling out of our driveway to return home, my dad called my phone. "Sis, go out your front door and look. There is a double rainbow over your house!"

Rushing out the front door, I looked up. A double rainbow. Another sign from God! I thought back to the rainbow that appeared above our son's home the day before my first chemo—a sign from God that he was with me. And now five months later, this! God was reminding me he was still in control! I knew he would get me through the storm . . . through the flood of treatments and pain yet to come.

God had brought me home after a long, hard journey. And he would be with me through whatever was yet to come. The rainbows reminded me he would carry me through this storm as he had Noah in the flood.

I am trusting you, Lord! You have given me strength and endurance. You have protected me from serious reactions and provided me with successful treatment and surgery. You are my protector and healer. This rainbow reminds me you are in control!

I have read articles teaching that rainbows are reminders of God's promises that he has not forgotten us. His promises have never failed. I knew he was with me at that moment, showing his presence in such a marvelous way. Both rainbows had been beautiful and unexpected—and reminded me how great our God is. And he made this double rainbow just today at this place for me! Praise God for his love!

Reflections

Here are some of my favorite Scriptures about rainbows.

And instantly I was in the Spirit, and I saw a throne in heaven and someone sitting on it. The one sitting on the throne was as brilliant as gemstones—like jasper and carnelian. And the glow of an emerald circled his throne like a rainbow.

— REVELATION 4:2–3

All around him was a glowing halo, like a rainbow shining in the clouds on a rainy day. This is what the glory of the Lord looked like to me.

— EZEKIEL 1:28

"When I send clouds over the earth, the rainbow will appear in the clouds, and I will remember my covenant with you and with all living creatures. Never again will the floodwaters destroy all life. When I see the rainbow in the clouds, I will remember the eternal covenant between God and every living creature on earth."

— GENESIS 9:14–16

There is victory in the seen and unseen victory in those things not yet seen. This cancer journey had been a huge, long-lasting battle. I didn't know when it would end, but the rainbow reminded me Jesus had already won the battle for me.

Now faith is the assurance (title deed, confirmation) of things hoped for (divinely guaranteed), and the evidence of things not seen [the conviction of their reality—faith comprehends as fact what cannot be experienced by the physical senses].

— Hebrews 11:1 AMP

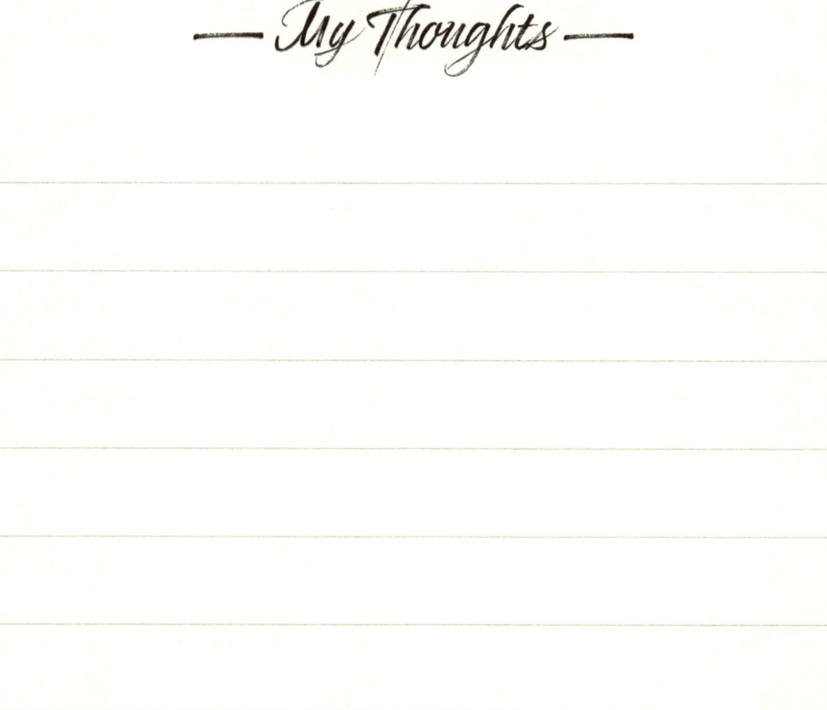

59

FOOTPRINTS

October 14, 2021. After six months in Texas with trips home only a few times, we were so excited to finally be back. We would return to MD Anderson for checkups every three months for a year and then for annual checkups for five years. I had radiation and chemo doctors in my hometown of Joplin, Missouri. The doctors at MD would follow my care and provide direction and assistance.

I was relaxed to be home but still needed a lot of healing—both physically and emotionally. The additional treatments would take ten months. I felt as if I were still in the ark, floating along and more than ready for the rain to stop and the waters to subside. I thought how eager Noah must have been to get off that ark. So far, I had ridden through the storm having tests, biopsies, six chemo treatments and their side effects, and a mastectomy.

I thought of the continuing storm. I understood it would be rough—thirty rounds of radiation and fourteen more rounds of chemo.

Although my surgery was healing and I could move my arm up and around, it quickly became stiff with inactivity. I also had some swelling under the arm that I prayed would not be long-term.

Although David, family, and friends continued their loving support, some days I felt so discouraged. I prayed daily for God's mercy. I gained strength from several cancer devotional books and wrote in my journals every day about my feelings.

Reflections

At one time we had a picture hanging on our wall showing footprints in the sand. The caption read, "When you see only one set of footprints, it's then that Jesus is carrying you!"

I pictured two pairs of footprints walking side by side. At one point there was only one pair. Jesus had been walking with me. I knew the change to one pair of prints meant Jesus had begun to carry me. On this day I felt as if I were starting to walk beside

God again. My prints were finally back in the sand! Praise the Lord!

Please know that whenever the going gets too difficult, Jesus will pick you up and carry you. Rest in his arms. Trust him. When you are ready, he will tenderly set you down on the sand but will always hold your hand. I encourage you to meditate on these Scriptures.

The Lord directs the steps of the godly. He delights in every detail of their lives. Though they stumble, they will never fall, for the Lord holds them by the hand.

— Psalm 37:23–24

"For I hold you by your right hand—I, the Lord your God. And I say to you, 'Don't be afraid. I am here to help you.'"

— Isaiah 41:13

"Don't be afraid, for I am with you. Don't be discouraged, for I am your God. I will strengthen you and help you. I will hold you up with my victorious right hand."

— Isaiah 41:10

I know the Lord is always with me. I will not be shaken, for he is right beside me.

— Psalm 16:8

My Thoughts

60

SHARING

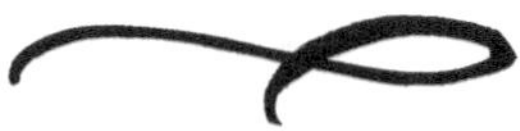

It took time for me to understand the realities of the mastectomy and the adjustments it would require. The medical team told me I may have a feeling of loss. Now I knew what they meant. I felt sad. My body did not feel normal. At times I didn't feel I was even in my own skin.

At this point, my mind still did not stay on track. In fact, sometimes my thought process was at zero! I had great difficulty expressing myself and was often unable to find the right words to complete a sentence.

My vision was blurred, and my eyes watered. My hands and feet still hurt from the neuropathy. The rash on one foot was still bad, with the skin peeling all the time. The nails on that foot had just lifted off and still didn't grow much. I was thankful some of the red sores were clearing up. The face rash was also better—I thought about trying a little makeup soon. I experienced less diarrhea but had been warned it would worsen when chemo treatments restarted.

I still cried a lot and had many sleepless nights—often ending up in the recliner or on the sofa trying to sleep.

I thought of the cautions I had received. "You will have chemo brain. . . . You sometimes won't be able to pull up a word. . . . You may have sadness from the loss." Now I was beginning to understand.

Loss. That word described so much of what I felt. Not being able to do whatever I wanted to do. Loss of so much time because of doctors' appointments, treatments, and feeling too sick to do anything. Loss of body parts and functions like feeling in fingers and feet, fingernails—and now, loss of a breast.

Reflections

Many cancer patients I visited with didn't want to talk about what they had been through. I desperately wanted to find out if my reactions and feelings were normal, but only a few would share with me how they had felt. Most post-cancer and now cancer-free would just say, "You'll get through it." I think I understand now why it was so difficult to talk about, and I don't fault them for that. Some shared they were past it and didn't want to relive it.

I believe it's so important for anyone on a cancer journey—or any journey of suffering—to know their feelings and experiences are normal, and I want to encourage and give hope to other cancer patients. As you read this devotional, I hope you will realize what you are feeling is normal. More importantly, I pray you will find hope and strength in God's Word and his love. And that someday you will be able to comfort others with the kind of comfort God is giving you!

I attended two cancer support groups in Texas, where I was encouraged to remain positive. I heard again and again, "Yes, that is how I felt. It is real!" Their honest sharing of feelings helped me know I was normal and could improve and get through the journey! Hope grew that I would not be stuck with chemo brain or painful skin and diarrhea. Someday I would be able to take long soaks in the tub or even long, warm showers. Someday I would feel more like myself. And so will you.

Pray that God will use your journey to enable you to comfort and help others. As you trust him, he will bring good from even the darkest of times.

And we know that God causes everything to work together for the good of those who love God and are called according to his purpose for them.

— ROMANS 8:28

All praise to God, the Father of our Lord Jesus Christ. God is our merciful Father and the source of all comfort. He comforts us in all our troubles so that we can comfort others. When they are troubled, we will be able to give them the same comfort God has given us.

— 2 CORINTHIANS 1:3–4

— *My Thoughts* —

61

CHOICES

October 15, 2021. I was busy doing *what* I could *when* I could. It was a wonderful feeling. We spent this day doing laundry, unpacking, and putting away all we had brought home from our six-month stay in Texas. I had a cold and prayed it would not turn into COVID. I worked slowly, and David helped a lot.

I was still very tired and weak but knew recovering from a major surgery took months, sometimes as long as a year. And in addition to the surgery, my body had experienced many dye tests, treatments, biopsies, and six rounds of chemo. It *should* be tired! The drugs had taken my blood counts below normal, and they had to rebuild. I had also had an amputation of a body part, and my chest needed more time to heal.

Sometimes I had feelings the amputated breast was still there—phantom pain. As a nurse, I had taken care of amputation patients who would say they still felt their removed body part, but I had never heard that about a breast. It was very strange to feel my nipple itching when it wasn't even there! (Ha ha.)

October 16. I went to see my local oncologist for the first time since surgery. The drain in my chest still wasn't ready to be removed. My blood work was good, but my potassium was slightly low, so I had to continue taking potassium every day. The doctor said we would begin chemo soon and radiation around Thanksgiving.

I also had a video consultation with my radiology doctor at MD Anderson. She said radiation should begin between six and twelve weeks post-op. I would have six weeks (thirty treatments) from neck to armpit. She explained the possible reactions: fatigue, skin rash, skin burns, and sore throat. A small percentage of radiation patients develop radiation pneumonia, which is treated with steroids.

Once again, my mind began to worry. The what-ifs haunted me. *Lord, please, please walk with me. Hold me safe in this storm!*

Reflections

Our hearts had been heavy that week because a lifelong friend had gone to his heavenly home after cancer. We know that life is short and years pass quickly. Life on this earth does end. God says heaven will be without pain or tears. We cannot know how truly wonderful it will be, but we long to be there at the end of our earthly lives. At the same time, it is easy to want to stay on earth to have more time here with our loved ones. Just before going to the cross, Jesus asked his Father that the cup be taken from him if possible. He knew where he was going, but I am sure he didn't want the horrific pain or to leave those he loved on earth. Is that why he cried and asked for it to pass? His prayer makes it all the more understandable that we grieve the loss of loved ones.

Jesus's death on the cross and his resurrection are also a reminder that we need to prepare for the day we leave earth. As believers, we need to ask God to help us accomplish his purpose for us here. We need to trust completely in his way, his plan, his timing. *What will I do with the days I have left? Will I serve the Lord . . . or will I live the days in fear?* Daily, even when we are feeling our worst, we must make those choices.

We all need to be sure of our destination when we leave earth. Jesus makes it so clear that the only way to heaven is through him. If you've never invited him into your life as your personal Lord and Savior, I urge you to make that choice. It's by far the most important decision you will ever make.

If you openly declare that Jesus is Lord and believe in your heart that God raised him from the dead, you will be saved. For it is by believing in your heart that you are made right with God, and it is by openly declaring your faith that you are saved.

— ROMANS 10:9–10

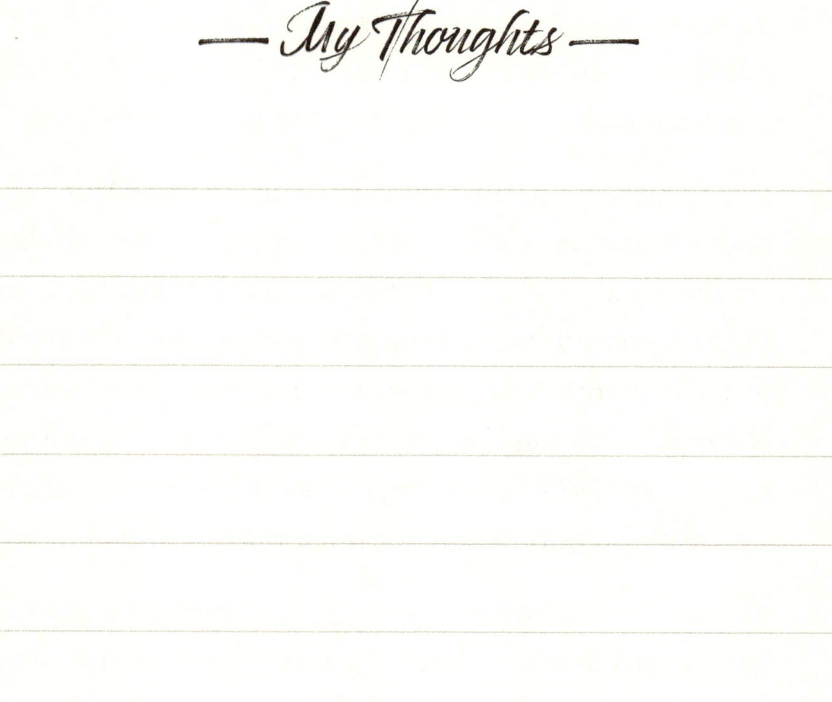

62

THE GOOD MOMENTS

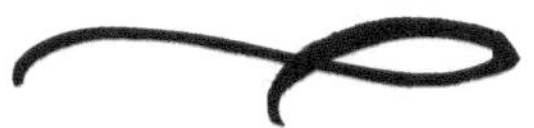

October 22, 2021. I was feeling good! And I was excited! We were headed to Tulsa for my niece Marylee's wedding! One of my first prayers at the beginning of treatment (and throughout all the treatments) was that I would finish the initial chemo and surgery and be well enough to attend her wedding. God had answered my prayer!

Thank you, Lord, for this day of health! I looked super good in my new dress. The outdoor wedding was beautiful, and the bride and groom were so happy. The dinner was relaxed, and the food delicious. I felt so blessed.

On the way home, we stopped in Miller, Missouri, at a pecan store. While there, I met the president of the breast cancer support group in Joplin. What a God thing! As usual, God's perfect timing. She promised to send me information about their meetings. I looked forward to getting together with the group when I was stronger and feeling better.

October 27. I had an appointment with the local radiology doctor. After our visit, she sent me to the radiation room for a CT of my organs. The man doing the CT said, "Okay, Vicki, we will be putting tattoos on you showing where the radiation should and shouldn't be done."

I had no idea this was coming. Wow! Those four small tattoo dots really did hurt! I can guarantee you, I will never want another tattoo of any kind. I do not want that pain again.

Lord, you are my strength. You are my power. Please heal me. Give me happiness and peace. Bring me positive thoughts to keep me happy even in the valleys of illness. Thank you, Lord, for holding my hand and helping me today.

October 28. The first of fourteen more chemo treatments today. The doctor said I should not have any additional numbness in my feet or hands—and no hair loss, so my hair should keep growing! I didn't have very much yet, but the little that had grown back eased the scalp tenderness and pain. I still wore hats for warmth. And I wore wigs to look like a woman!

Before the infusion came lab work and a visit with the doctor. Everything was a go for the treatment. My nurse was sweet and prayed with me first thing. They gave me Benadryl again, which made me very drowsy. I felt so drugged again. All went well. I was so sleepy, they wheelchaired me out to the car.

More treatments ahead. More sickness. More what-ifs. *Lord, please keep your hand on me. Walk with me. Extend your mighty right hand toward me, and hold me up!*

Reflections

Walking through a breast cancer journey brings much pain, sickness, fear, and confusion. It takes your time, your energy. It keeps you away from many or all of your daily routines and activities. But in looking back, I realize more than ever the value of recognizing the bright spots along the way—big and small—and thanking God for them. Buying a special dress and traveling to my niece's wedding was one of the big bright spots. Meeting the president of the Joplin support group—another blessing from God. Then good blood work so my infusions could begin . . . and no reactions during the infusion that day. My hair growing back. All good. I knew I needed to focus on the improvements—even small ones. I needed to focus on the 90 percent chance of no cancer return—not the 10 percent chance of return.

That's not an easy thing to do, but I encourage you to try. Thank God for every good or encouraging thing.

Tell others about the good. Write about the good in your journal. Think about the good.

And now, dear brothers and sisters, one final thing. Fix your thoughts on what is true, and honorable, and right, and pure, and lovely, and admirable. Think about things that are excellent and worthy of praise.... Then the God of peace will be with you.

— Philippians 4:8–9

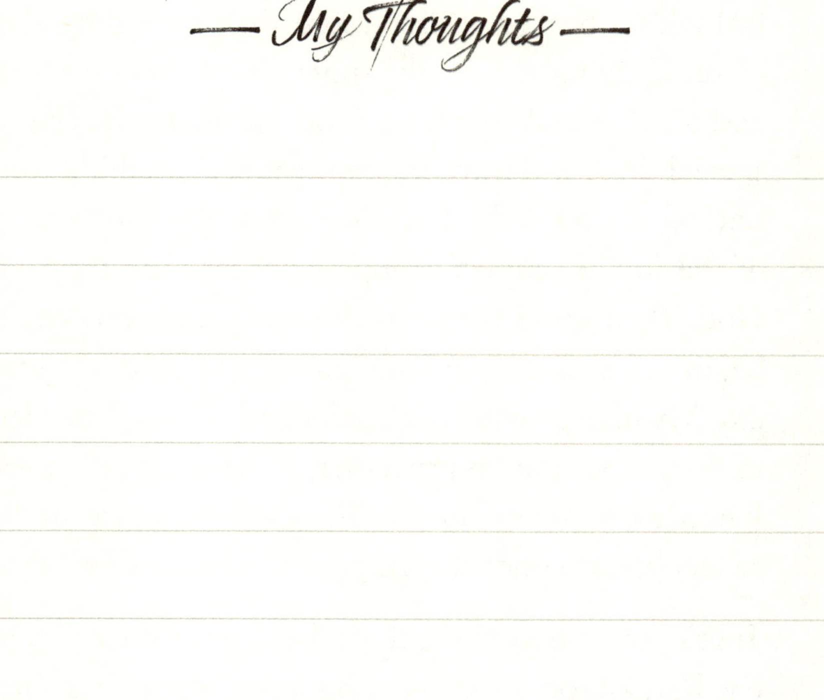

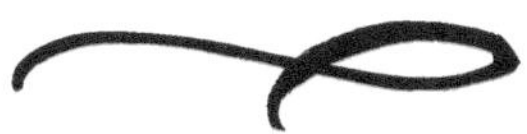

PRAY FOR OTHERS

October 29, 2021. I was super tired from the infusion. I took something for nausea but still didn't eat much. The metal taste lingered in my mouth. I knew I was able to endure the treatments only through God's strength. Prayers were holding me up!

November 2. A new month had begun. Colorful leaves were falling! My labs showed that my platelet count was critically low, which could cause bleeding internally or from my gums or skin. That's one reason I was so tired. I needed to watch for signs of bleeding. My potassium was still low as well, so I would continue taking it by mouth and eating lots of bananas.

November 4. I was a little stronger but was having some bone pain, along with being constipated. I began to think about decorating for Christmas. In the past, I usually had all my decorations up by November 1. I decided to put up fewer decorations—not only because of the strength needed to put them up but also thinking ahead to the strength needed to take them down! I didn't know how I may be feeling by then. I began by putting out a few table decorations.

Since I knew firsthand how hard chemo is, I prayed daily for everyone I knew who had cancer. That list was growing as either I just heard about others' diagnoses or people contacted me asking for prayer. I so appreciated the way family and friends were encouraging me, and I wanted to do that for others.

November 10. I was very tired and dizzy and experiencing more numbness in my fingers and feet. Although I pushed hard to eat, I still didn't manage to get much down. On the positive side, I was beginning to grow eyebrows again, and more and more hair was appearing on my head! People loved to touch it and feel the softness.

Lord, I want to be healthy. I want to live and help others on this earth. I want to see my grandkids succeed and be faithful to the Lord. Whatever lies ahead of me today, please give me your peace, your strength, and your love to get me through.

One way the Lord encouraged me was through worship at our church—hearing people around me singing. *Praise be to our Lord for his help in enduring this journey!*

Reflections

As I mentioned, I was focusing more and more on praying for others with cancer. I wanted God to use me—even during this journey, maybe *especially* during this journey. I found comfort in encouraging others and praying for them. I wanted to be serving God any way I could, and he was making that possible. I thought often of this verse I've pointed out before.

All praise to God, the Father of our Lord Jesus Christ. God is our merciful Father and the source of all comfort. He comforts us in all our troubles so that we can comfort others. When they are troubled, we will be able to give them the same comfort God has given us.

— 2 Corinthians 1:3–4

Even on the days you don't feel like it, I encourage you to pray for others. Maybe sometimes it's just whispering their names. God promises his children to bring good from everything, and this was one good I could see even at this point in my journey.

Carry one another's burdens and in this way you will fulfill the requirements of the law of Christ [that is, the law of Christian love].

— Galatians 6:2 AMP

I urge you, first of all, to pray for all people. Ask God to help them; intercede on their behalf, and give thanks for them.

— 1 TIMOTHY 2:1

— *My Thoughts* —

64

GOD HAS A
PURPOSE FOR YOU

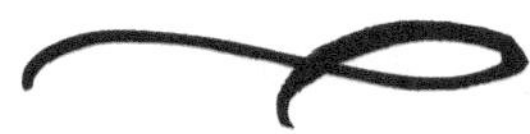

November 18. Labs before my second infusion showed a terrific rebound in my platelets. However, they decided to be cautious and lower the dosage of this infusion.

November 19. My heart was very sad. My Aunt Jeannine had died from cancer. When she had been ill for only a couple of months, it had reached the point they could no longer treat her. It is always so sad to say those final good-byes, but we found great comfort in knowing she was with Jesus.

The weekend was busy, and I was feeling better than after the previous infusion. Praise God! We would have family with us for the funeral.

November 22. Aunt Jeannine's funeral service was good. Our family enjoyed lunch together at the church. We would all miss her.

November 23. My first radiation, the first of six weeks of daily treatments. My platelets were still a little low but coming up. Potassium was still low.

November 24. I received a call at eight this morning that sent me straight to the hospital for a potassium infusion. Apparently, this week's chemo had dropped my potassium to a dangerous level—1.6.

I was crying when I arrived at the hospital. The nurse prayed with me and calmed me down. I had already had so many potassium infusions—along with taking it daily by mouth. For months now, I had taken so many medications. I didn't like how they made me feel. But even when this happened, I knew God was holding on to my body. *Lord, I pray there is not permanent damage to my major organs.*

November 25. Thanksgiving Day! A friend brought us lunch. What a blessing! I was so tired I could hardly walk up and down our stairs without stopping every other step. Still, my heart raced out of control. We so appreciated the lunch. God is good.

Reflections

So many ups and downs. I was reminded that we are all mortal beings. When we belong to Christ, we have the promise of a heavenly eternal life after we die. We can rejoice for that and live in that hope. *But*—I was not ready to leave earth. I was not ready to leave my family—I longed to stay with them a longer time. So . . . I determined to stand firm in my hope for God's healing from the cancer.

God is the giver of life. He knows the days of our lives. We all have a time to be born and a time to die. Whatever time God has planned for me, I want to use it living a life pleasing to him.

Lord, you have a plan for my life, so please let me be used for your purpose.

It is my own eager expectation and hope, that [looking toward the future] I will not disgrace myself nor be ashamed in anything, but that with courage and the utmost freedom of speech, even now as always, Christ will be magnified and exalted in my body, whether by life or by death.

— PHILIPPIANS 1:20 AMP

Never lagging behind in diligence; aglow in the Spirit, enthusiastically serving the Lord; constantly rejoicing in hope [because of our confidence in

Christ], steadfast and patient in distress, devoted to prayer [continually seeking wisdom, guidance, and strength].

— ROMANS 12:11–12 AMP

— My Thoughts —

65

EYES ON JESUS

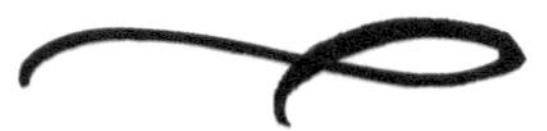

November 29, 2021. I had my third radiation treatment. So far, I was not burning, but super tired. The radiology doctor gave the go-ahead for the treatment but told me to continue watching for bleeding since my blood counts were still very low.

December 1. It had been eight months since my cancer diagnosis. So much had happened during that time. On this day I saw my oncologist in the morning and had blood drawn. Praise the Lord! Although my labs were still low, they had come up!

I was feeling good. I had done a little Christmas shopping, but we were not buying many gifts. Of course, we bought for our grandchildren.

Lord, all I can really do is ask you for help to get me through chemo, radiation, and healing from my mastectomy.

December 2. More radiation. I tried to do what I could to keep living, but that was hard when I felt so bad. And fear of the future kept robbing me of peace. I was sad because I had cancer. I cried easily from all the drugs. I feared the drugs, the pain, and the what-ifs concerning my future.

I began to prepare myself for the treatment. *Please help me not bleed or burn. Lord, I am in your hands. Hold me up to live!*

As I lay on the radiation table, I visualized my powerful God looking down from heaven, reaching his mighty right hand down to me and holding me up. I knew the best way to get through these hard days of fear and treatment was to see God walking with me!

That night we went to a Christmas program at Ozark Christian College with some friends. I was thankful to celebrate Jesus's birth and praise him for his love. Several friends at the program asked how I was doing. My reply to each one was, "It's been a hard journey, and I have had many side effects. God's help and prayers of friends have kept me going."

December 3. We attended a beautiful Christmas musical with my parents at their church. It was a wonderful time to think of Jesus and his love for us as he came to earth.

Although I was very tired, I pushed myself through to enjoy the Christmas music. It was difficult to get comfortable, though, because my chest was getting very red, tender, and painful. I was taking pain pills often and kept the area swathed with lotion.

Reflections

Do you sometimes feel as if the pain will never stop? As if your life will never again be normal? I had many of those thoughts, and I never found a "quick fix" for that. But I did learn that I would drown in the suffering if I did not keep my eyes on Jesus. That's why I visualized him looking down at me on the radiation table, reaching out to me with his love and strength. That's why I would envision the single pair of footsteps in the sand, knowing that through the worst times, Jesus was carrying me.

Jesus loves you. He cares. He will not leave you. And he will be with you every step of the journey.

As for me, I look to the Lord for help. I wait confidently for God to save me, and my God will certainly hear me.

— Micah 7:7

Yet I am confident I will see the Lord's goodness while I am here in the land of the living.

— PSALM 27:13

Yet I still belong to you; you hold my right hand.

— PSALM 73:23

— *My Thoughts* —

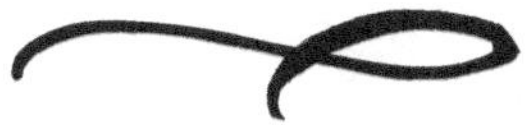

HOPING IN JESUS

December 15. I was halfway done with the thirty rounds of radiation (one every weekday). And I was burning. These radiation burns made me more aware of what hell will be like for those who don't receive Jesus as their Savior. I can tell you, you don't want to go there! I don't think we can even imagine how much pain there will be. For eternity.

Praise God that Jesus paid the price so we can spend eternity with him instead.

> But God showed his great love for us by sending Christ to die for us while we were still sinners. And since we have been made right in God's sight by the blood of Christ, he will certainly save us from God's condemnation. For since our friendship with God was restored by the death of his Son while we were still his

enemies, we will certainly be saved through the life of his Son. So now we can rejoice in our wonderful new relationship with God because our Lord Jesus Christ has made us friends of God.

— ROMANS 5:8–11

Unlike eternity in hell, praise God my time of suffering from burns was temporary. Here on earth I was blessed to get some medicine for them. And I knew the pain would end when I'd healed from the radiation. It might get worse before it got better, but I knew there was an end in sight. That gave me hope! Once again, I focused on *hope*.

December 20. Oh, my! The burning from radiation was worse, and I was more tired and weak. I looked sick in my eyes and face. I still could not wear makeup, and my nails continued to break off in the quick and peel. More pain. The rash on my feet continued to hurt as well. Most nights I was sleeping in my recliner or on the sofa with only a light cover over me. I couldn't stand anything touching the burns. I was so restless and fearful, and the tears kept flowing.

Lord, lift me up.

At night David read me Scriptures. Many nights he even sang to me, giving me hope of a better tomorrow. Although the pain and weakness continued, I was grateful to wake up each morning and have another day of hope.

Reflections

During your journey, I am sure you have had days similar to the ones I just described. Remember, that is normal. You will have those days, but what you do with them is up to you. As you have read again and again in this devotional book, I struggled. I questioned. I feared. I cried. But I learned that placing my hope in Jesus . . . trusting him . . . was what I needed to make it through.

Above, I described some of the ways I was able to cling to hope. Focusing on Scripture. Reading it, praying it, saying it aloud. And listening to music filled with hope in Jesus. Whether you can carry a tune or not, when you are able, sing those words! And, of course, pray. Just talk to Jesus. Say his name. Let him fill you with hope.

Here are some Scriptures to look up. Read them aloud. Meditate on them. Personalize them. Pray them. You can have hope! Live with that hope as Jesus carries you through the journey.

Having hope will give you courage. You will be protected and will rest in safety.

— JOB 11:18

So be strong and courageous, all you who put your hope in the Lord!

— Psalm 31:24

Let us hold fast the confession of our hope without wavering, for he who promised is faithful.

— Hebrews 10:23 ESV

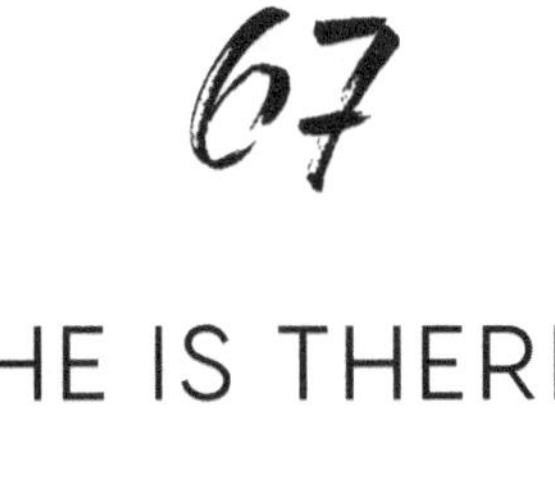

67

HE IS THERE

December 20–23, 2021. Because of Christmas, only four radiation treatments this week instead of the usual five! Praise the Lord!

The burns hurt so badly I still could not wear any clothing on the top half of my body. Since we had company, I laid a cotton t-shirt over my shoulder or sometimes cut the right side out of a t-shirt, allowing my left side to still be covered. It was winter, and I was cold! Pain pills made me even more tired than I already was from the chemo, low blood counts, and radiation burns.

Even with all this, our home was filled with joy. Son Shon and his family and my brother, Jeff, and his family were there for Christmas. It was wonderful to have them with us (fourteen people)—and they did all the cooking! Our home was filled with fun, games, laughter, and gifts!

Although I still went to the hospital daily for treatments (except Christmas Day) and was very tired, I was able to enjoy the family time together.

My mind was clearer and I was gradually feeling better. But when I went to radiation that week, I was overwhelmed with fear as I lay there with the machines going all around me. I focused on Jesus. *You are my God, who reaches down your mighty right hand and lifts me up.*

December 24. All of us went to the Christmas Eve gathering at our church, then to my parents' church for their service. After, we all went out to dinner. I was doing fair physically that day but was filled with so many mixed emotions. I cried from pain and fear. But I also cried with gratitude that the kids were there and helped me so much.

December 25. Christmas Day. Our daughter-in-law Michelle cooked dinner. We enjoyed every bite! A friend dropped by with a tray filled with cookies. I was so blessed with friends providing gifts, food, and prayers. All the family left for home the next day.

December 27–31. Five radiation treatments this week and the last four the first week in January. More burns.

Reflections

Lord, how can I take the pain? Lord, are you nearby? Do you hear my cry?

This was a difficult journey I had never dreamed I'd be on. *How do I hang on to God?* All around me were family and friends, yet sometimes I felt so alone. I couldn't feel their presence even though they were there. And sometimes I could not feel the Lord's presence. But his Word promises me he will never leave me nor forsake me, and I know he always keeps his promises. So even when I couldn't "feel" him, he was there.

I encourage you to remember that as well. Cling to his promises. Know that when things are the most difficult, he is carrying you (one set of footprints in the sand). And he is holding your hand *all* the time.

He knows you are hurting—and he cares. He will get you through this. He will never leave you.

"What's more, I am with you, and I will protect you wherever you go. One day I will bring you back to this land. I will not leave you until I have finished giving you everything I have promised you."

— Genesis 28:15

"Do not be afraid or discouraged, for the Lord will personally go ahead of you. He will be with you; he will neither fail you nor abandon you."

— Deuteronomy 31:8

"And be sure of this: I am with you always, even to the
end of the age."

— Matthew 28:20

— *My Thoughts* —

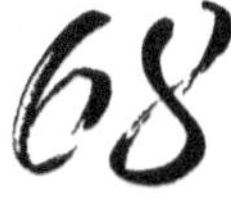

PRAISES!

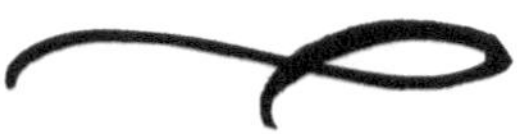

December 20, 2021. It was time for my fourth chemo infusion in the second round of treatments. Except for potassium, my labs were good. Praise the Lord! I was cleared for my treatment.

This was also the day to begin direct radiation to my right chest and armpit. That left me with hot red burns all over the right side around to my back. *I do not want to do this again in my life, so, Lord, I ask you to please heal me forever!*

Good news. Definitely a praise the Lord! The day before, I had noticed that I had hair on my legs and under my arms—and more on my head each day. It had taken four months to begin growing after finishing the first type of chemo in August. My wigs and hats had been cute but became hot and irritating to my sensitive head. Hopefully, by May I would have enough hair to stop wearing wigs.

At this point, my new hair was pretty and curly—and stuck out every which way! David was so happy not to have a bald wife anymore. He loved to touch and comb my new hair.

I was very thankful for friends who had provided meals through the December treatments. And for the cards, gifts, flowers, text messages, and calls of encouragement.

Through all the pain and fears and sickness, there was always something to be thankful for. And I felt so much better when I took time to focus on those blessings! I determined to praise the Lord with my whole heart, to praise his holy name. Even though it was hard to praise him when I felt so alone and sick, I would not stop. Sometimes I praised him by listening to—or singing—"How Great Thou Art." That helped me focus on his love and on my many blessings instead of on the fear and pain.

> I will praise you as long as I live, lifting up my hands to you in prayer.
>
> — PSALM 63:4

Reflections

I encourage you to focus on your blessings—and praise God, because they all come from him! Meditate on these Scriptures. Then take some time to write down ways God has blessed you through this journey. You may even want to add to that list every day!

Whatever is good and perfect is a gift coming down to us from God our Father, who created all the lights in the heavens.

— JAMES 1:17

Let all that I am praise the Lord; with my whole heart, I will praise his holy name.

— PSALM 103:1

All praise to God, the Father of our Lord Jesus Christ, who has blessed us with every spiritual blessing in the heavenly realms because we are united with Christ.

— EPHESIANS 1:3

Then I will praise God's name with singing, and I will honor him with thanksgiving.

— PSALM 69:30

Be thankful in all circumstances, for this is God's will for you who belong to Christ Jesus.

— 1 Thessalonians 5:18

— My Thoughts —

69

OVERCOMING FEAR

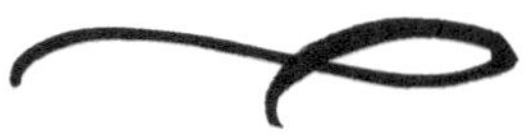

January 2022. A new year! My faith and fears had been up and down throughout this journey.

Lord, I know you have provided comfort, and you have given me strength and brought peace to me often. Lord, you have provided rest and health many, many days from April 2021 until today. Although my fears and faith go up and down, I come before you to praise you for all you have already done.

You died for me. You love me and made heaven for my future life. Lord, I pray and ask forgiveness for my weakness and fear of sickness and death and for my fear of leaving my family. I pray for many more healthy years but also for peace, health, confidence, and life. Protect my body from the next chemo treatments, radiation, and all cancer.

The cancer is all cut out, so why do I fear? I fear the effects of chemo and radiation. My burns hurt and are so bad. It's hard not to fear damage to my liver, lungs, and heart. Only by your hand will I be safe and have no damage. Only you can heal this serious treatment! Lord, forgive me for my weakness. Keep your Word in my heart so I will remember your greatness.

I knew there was no temptation not common to man, and my greatest temptation at that time was fear. But God promised he would provide a way of escape.

> No temptation has overtaken you that is not common to man. God is faithful, and he will not let you be tempted beyond your ability, but with the temptation he will also provide the way of escape, that you may be able to endure it.
>
> — 1 CORINTHIANS 10:13 ESV

I am overwhelmed with fear and sorrow. Lord, I ask you to please remove all these feelings and bring me peace and joy as you make me well. Pull me through this cancer journey. And, Lord, please stay in control.

> Don't worry about anything; instead, pray about everything. Tell God what you need, and thank him for all he has done. Then you will experience God's peace, which exceeds anything we can understand.

His peace will guard your hearts and minds as you live in Christ Jesus.

— Philippians 4:6–7

Fear is difficult to control and understand. I repeated these words again and again:

- I will finish (six more months of chemo—ten infusions).
- I will stay strong.
- I will be joyful.
- I will be healed.
- I will trust in you.
- Lord, you are my strength!

Reflections

Anxiety can make you physically and mentally ill. I encourage you to go to God daily—and some days hourly—for peace. The Bible teaches we are to be content in all circumstances. That is easy when everything is right and going well. However, when life is hard . . . when it is turned upside down with death, sickness, pain, loss of hope for tomorrow . . . fear is real, and the only way to peace is Jesus.

For God has not given us a spirit of fear and timidity, but of power, love, and self-discipline.

— 2 Timothy 1:7

I prayed to the LORD, and he answered me. He freed me from all my fears.

— PSALM 34:4

70

REACHING OUT

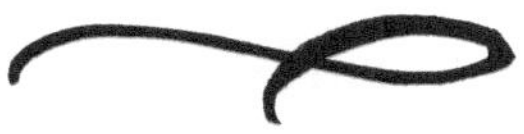

January 6, 2022. For a while now, I had been focusing on people and finding ways to encourage them. I called, texted friends with birthdays, wrote happy notes, and sent gifts for special occasions. I prayed for and called new cancer patients. Doing this probably blessed me even more than it did them.

I was walking every day to get some exercise, and I was beginning to cook some. One of my first attempts was making chili. Taking my first bite, I looked at David and said, "This is terrible." He laughed and agreed. We threw it out! I still had some metal taste, so my cooking was not yet ready to be shared with anyone.

Back to the present. This was a special day. My last radiation treatment! They had me ring the bell for finishing another round of treatment! The radiation had continued for six weeks with a total of thirty treatments! Burns, blisters, and pain. Sleepless nights and exhaustion. Not an easy journey. But God, again, had kept me safe with no major problems. I continued praying that my internal organs would not be damaged and that healthy cells would rebuild quickly.

January 15. I was doing pretty well. The scabs were off, and my skin was healing. With less pain, I was able to wear a t-shirt. There was still some swelling under my arm.

It was snowing! Praise the Lord that he covered my sins and made me whiter than snow. *Lord, give me peace as white as snow.* It is so important to look for God's glory in everything around us. The glory of God is always with us. That day I saw it in the birds of the air . . . the snow on the ground . . . and the peace in my heart!

January 18. Lots of tests. Bone density, ECHO, EKG, aorta scan, and an ultrasound of my heart—all at Mercy Hospital in Joplin. The reports were sent to MD Anderson and to my heart doctor in Texas. I was excited to learn that my ECHO was normal—even after all the chemo. All the tests were normal for my age and situation. Praise the Lord!

January 20. My fifth chemo infusion—only nine to go!

Reflections

I learned that reaching out to others with texts, calls, notes, and more helped *me* so much. First, because that's what God wants us to do.

Don't look out only for your own interests, but take an interest in others, too.

— PHILIPPIANS 2:4

Share each other's burdens, and in this way obey the law of Christ.

— GALATIANS 6:2

Therefore, whenever we have the opportunity, we should do good to everyone—especially to those in the family of faith.

— GALATIANS 6:10

Second, I learned from experience that as we do what God is calling us to do and focus on being kind to others, our spirits are lifted. We are more fully focused on Jesus and on others and a little less focused on our own suffering and problems.

The same holds true when we look for God's glory in everything around us. That particular day I saw his glory in the snow and was reminded of his love and what he did for me on the cross. I saw it in his creation—the birds. And I felt it in my heart—the peace he gave me. Where do you see his glory right now?

♡ — *My Thoughts* —

71

NO MATTER WHAT

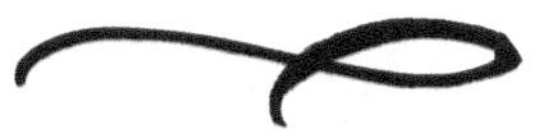

January 26, 2022. I felt overwhelmed. My mom had been sick and hadn't completely recovered yet. We were both still so sad about losing my aunt. My burns, although better, were not yet healed. And the following week David would be having a knee replacement.

I needed strength from God!

Lord, are you testing my faith? Why so many health issues? Lord, I trust you. I cling to you, Lord, to provide strength and healing. Lord, please bind Satan from our home, family, and health.

January 30. I was feeling very good. My burned skin was almost healed, and I was pressing on!

I knew I would have to take an anti-estrogen pill for five to ten years. However, because of the many side effects it could cause, I asked the doctors to give me a little more time to heal before I started to take it.

January had been a difficult month. The pain had been the worst of any during this journey. I had experienced more fear than ever and still was concerned about the possibility of radiation damage to my lungs and heart. I had gone into the radiation treatments thinking they would be easy—no one had wanted to tell me the extent of pain and suffering. If you will be going through radiation, I urge you to stand firm. Lean on God each day. Spend time in meditation and rest when you can—don't try to do all your normal daily activities. And count down the days, remembering there is an end in sight. When lying in the X-ray machine, pray. Say a verse you chose before going into the room. Lean on the Lord all afternoon and evening.

I was praying for strength and a positive mind. For more faith to believe for healing and to press on in life. Since I couldn't go anyplace because of the cold weather and because I wasn't feeling well yet, I spent my days sending cards, doing puzzles, praying, and reading God's Word. We were also preparing for David's knee replacement in a couple of days. He would have a second surgery six weeks later.

Reflections

I've talked about this before, but it can't be said too many times. No matter what you are going through … no matter how bad things look or how terrible you may feel … place your hope in the Lord. Talk to him. Meditate on his Word. Focus on his love.

Here are a few of many, many Scriptures filled with hope—you may have others that speak hope to you. Write them down. Pray them. Speak them aloud. Stay strong as you trust God. Hope in God's power and strength to heal and bring you through.

"The Lord himself will fight for you. Just stay calm."

— Exodus 14:14

The Lord is my shepherd; I have all that I need. He lets me rest in green meadows; he leads me beside peaceful streams. He renews my strength. He guides me along right paths, bringing honor to his name. Even when I walk through the darkest valley, I will not be afraid, for you are close beside me. Your rod and your staff protect and comfort me. You prepare a feast for me in the presence of my enemies. You honor me by anointing my head with oil. My cup overflows with blessings. Surely your goodness and unfailing love will pursue me all the days of my life, and I will live in the house of the Lord forever.

— Psalm 23

May the God of hope fill you with all joy and peace in believing, so that by the power of the Holy Spirit you may abound in hope.

— Romans 15:13 ESV

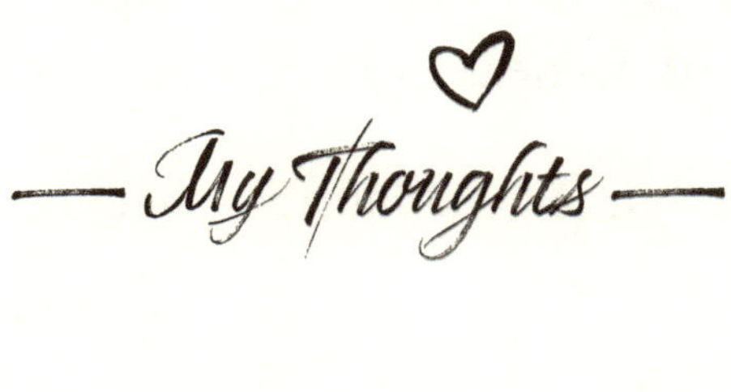

ONE SOURCE OF HOPE

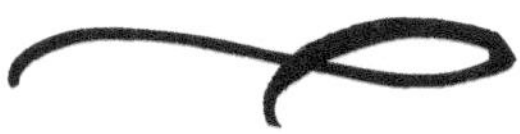

February 1–2, 2022. David had a total knee replacement. I was praying for his healing as well as mine. I knew we must walk in hope.

> I pray that God, the source of hope, will fill you completely with joy and peace because you trust in him. Then you will overflow with confident hope through the power of the Holy Spirit.
>
> — Romans 15:13

We wanted to live with joy in every circumstance. We had walked bravely during the difficult situations of the previous nine months. Day by day, we found peace only in Christ. We tried to be content in circumstances as we would continue the next six months with chemo every three weeks. We were thankful for my local doctor, as well as my doctor at MD Anderson, for helping us along the journey.

When I became anxious, I prayed the fear would be replaced with hope and I would be content.

I have learned how to be content with whatever I have.

— PHILIPPIANS 4:11

After you have suffered a little while, he will restore, support, and strengthen you, and he will place you on a firm foundation.

— 1 PETER 5:10

I praise you, Lord, that most of the chemo is behind me. I thank you that my surgery is healed and the radiation is done. I ask that the next treatments don't give me problems. Lord, please protect my organs and prevent internal bleeding. May my blood counts come up and my tiredness become less. Give me strength, Lord. I long to exercise again at the Y and be stronger.

May my emotions become more stable, with less fear and crying. Make my mind more alert, and may I have less chemo brain!

Lord, keep my parents' health stable and strong. I lift David up for his knee surgeries to have no problems. I pray he will heal well so he can walk better.

I pray we can soon enjoy time together with friends! Thank you, Lord, for your love.

Reflections

Like me, you may be experiencing many ups and downs—both physically and emotionally—throughout this journey. It's important to talk to God about the valleys as well as the mountaintops. At times you are probably experiencing fear . . . doubt . . . frustration . . . and maybe even anger. Jesus understands that and is always there for you. He is the one who can quiet the fear . . . restore your faith .. . calm the frustration . . . and take away the anger. He is your hope, so I encourage you to freely talk to him about all you are feeling—he knows anyhow! And he wants to help. Not only does he *want to help*, but he is also your *source of help*. Sometimes he will work through other people to help you, but *he* is always your source.

Here is an example of the way I prayed during some of the low times: *Greater is he that is in me than he that is in the world. God will take down this wall. Lord, I know you have already won the battle. You have beaten Satan. God, give me strength, courage, and peace. Lord, hold me steadfast with peace and rest. Help me fight to recover! Don't let stress or sadness depress my immune system. Help me remember that you are for me, and I have a reason to live. My hand clings to your right hand, Lord. Reach down your mighty right hand and lift me up out of the pit! Praise the Lord!*

We also pray that you will be strengthened with all his glorious power so you will have all the endurance and patience you need. May you be filled with joy, always thanking the Father.

— COLOSSIANS 1:11–12

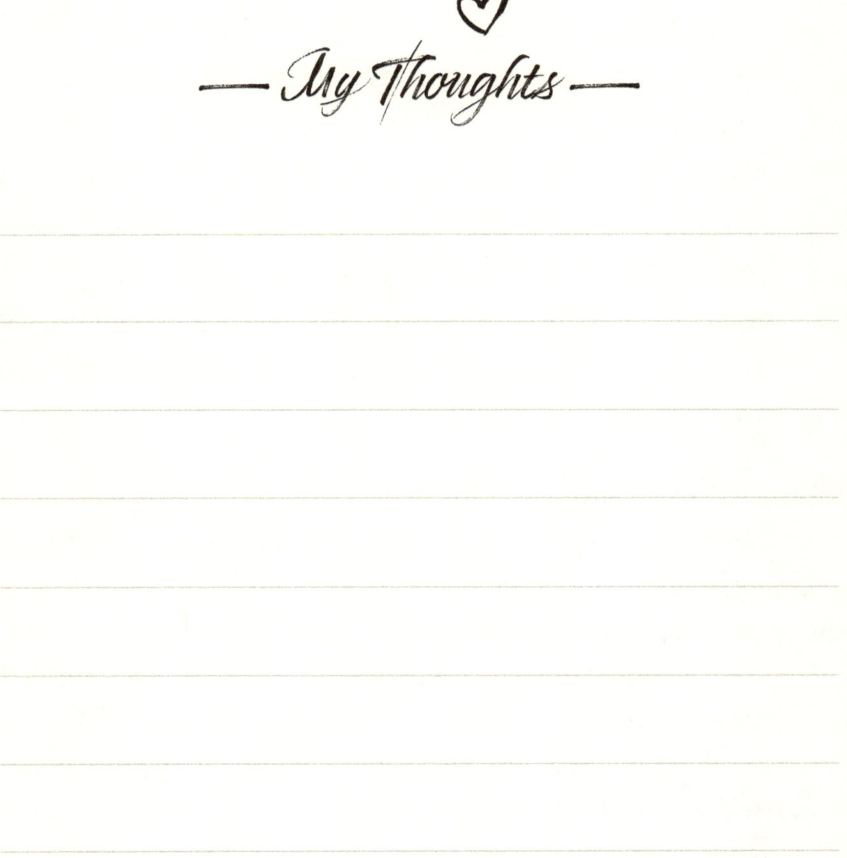

73

BUSY CAN BE GOOD

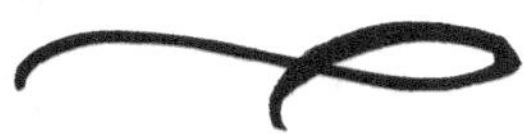

February 10, 2022. It was time for my sixth infusion. My friend Marcia took me. David was still not able to drive because of his knee surgery, and I would be too sleepy from the drugs to drive home. Always looking for a way to show my appreciate to the medical team, I took them a big basket filled with Valentine goodies. The treatment went as normal.

February 14. David was doing well from his knee replacement. I praised the Lord because my burns from radiation were finally healed—all that remained were some redness in the incision area and some swelling under my arm. I continued praying that God would protect my internal organs.

We tried to stay busy during this healing time for both of us. We did 1,000-piece jigsaw puzzles. I did a little cooking, but it still wasn't very good! David had at-home PT every week. And we enjoyed the snow all week from inside the house.

February 17. The radiology doctor released me! I did a little grocery shopping after my appointment with her. I so enjoyed going to the store, even though I had only enough strength to buy a few things at a time. I looked forward to the day I could do some real shopping again!

Praise God! Since I had finished the radiation treatments, now I had only one treatment (chemo) at a time! Wow! That was wonderful! My blood work was holding steady, and my hair was still growing! Praise God!

"The joy of the Lord is your strength!"

— Nehemiah 8:10

Lord, lift me up through my weakness, fear, sadness. Lord, help me to eat better! May I have less finger and foot numbness. Lord, please bring my blood counts up more with the next labs. Help me not to be so tired. May I have confidence and positive thoughts. Lord, let me see the light of health. Lord, make my mom stronger and help David walk with no pain. Lord, give me peace and direction for my healthcare.

February 22. My prayer journal was growing each month with entries about more friends who had cancer. I prayed every day for the specific needs of each one. (Even as I am writing this book, those numbers continue to grow—

many I am praying for are people I don't even know!) I was spending much time with the Lord in prayer.

The Lord is good to those who depend on him, to those who search for him.

— LAMENTATIONS 3:25

Reflections

I encourage you to stay busy doing positive things as much as possible throughout your journey. Some days you may not be able to, but do it whenever you can—even if you have to give yourself a special nudge. And whenever possible, include another person.

David and I enjoy doing jigsaw puzzles, so that was one of our "keep busy" activities. Maybe you and a friend or your spouse could play board games or card games. If you are a craft person, keep that going—even if just a few minutes at a time. Of course, walking is always good.

I also encourage you to pray for others—whatever their needs. Send cards and notes of encouragement. God wants to use you. Allow his love to flow through you to others.

"You are the light of the world—like a city on a hilltop that cannot be hidden. No one lights a lamp and then puts it under a basket. Instead, a lamp is placed on a stand, where it gives light to everyone in the house. In the same way, let your good deeds shine out for all to see, so that everyone will praise your heavenly Father."

— Matthew 5:14–16

♡

— *My Thoughts* —

74

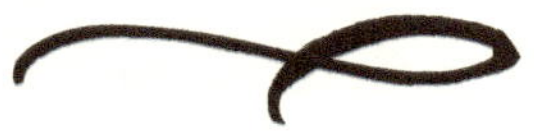

HIS GRACE IS ALL WE NEED

March 1, 2022. I played pickleball for the first time in ten months! Although I had a great time, I shouldn't have rushed getting back to it. There was too much possibility of being hit at my infusion port site. Also, I was still somewhat weak, and my platelet count was not much above 100. My doctor in Texas confirmed I shouldn't play until I had finished the chemo treatments. So, no more pickleball for a while. I didn't want to use all my blood and energy for working out—I needed everything for healing.

I was able to walk as long as I didn't overdo it. I usually went three to four times a week, two to three miles at a time.

I had my first haircut since my journey had begun in April 2021. Almost a full year! It wasn't long yet but needed to be shaped. My beautician would not let me pay her. She had been doing my hair for twenty-six years and had blessed me with Scriptures and prayer throughout this journey. *Lord, please bless her and others who serve you and help others.*

On this particular day, I told myself to focus on joy, love, peace, and faith. *Lord, I lift my hands to you for power from your Holy Spirit to flow through me.*

Unfailing love surrounds those who trust the Lord.

— Psalm 32:10

Reflections

I was feeling very contemplative. I thought about how important it was to stay in God's Word. If my heart became hard, I wouldn't hear his Word. Then I wouldn't feel compassion for others. I would serve God only half-heartedly. *Lord, how open is my heart? Am I serving with a heart of love—or am I serving just to get by? Where is my heart, oh Lord? How can I minister to others when I am so weak and sick?*

As I pondered these questions, I began to realize I could minister even in my weakness. I was ministering by accepting the many gifts gratefully . . . sending cards . . . sharing the abundance of food people blessed us with. Yes, I could serve even in this deep, dark time of my own sickness. I could pray for others and, when able, call them with encouragement.

My serving has been limited during this time of sickness. But, Lord, may my heart be happy and my face shine. Lord, I am thankful you have helped me find my serving heart. I pray my service will be acceptable to you, Lord. I want to show you and your love to the world.

The apostle Paul sought God about a "thorn in his flesh." He tells us about the Lord's response.

Each time he said, "My grace is all you need. My power works best in weakness." So now I am glad to boast about my weaknesses, so that the power of Christ can work through me.

— 2 CORINTHIANS 12:9

And the Lord reminded me that he wanted me to make the most of every opportunity, especially with unbelievers.

Conduct yourself with wisdom in your interactions with outsiders (non-believers), make the most of each opportunity [treating it as something precious].

— COLOSSIANS 4:5 AMP

I encourage you to ponder some of the same questions. Ask God to show you the ways you are already serving him. Ask him to fill your heart with his love and compassion for others and show you more ways you can reach out, even during your difficult journey. Remember, his grace is all you need. His power works best in our weaknesses.

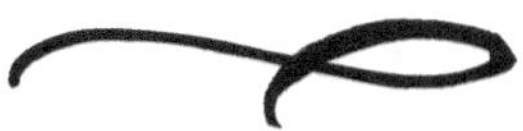

75

GOD HAS GONE BEFORE YOU

March 3, 2022. Seventh infusion. Seven down and seven to go. Praise the Lord!

Before the treatment, I met with my local doctor and asked him about post-treatment damage, especially to my lungs and heart. He said damage *afterward* was not likely. More likely, the issues would arise *during* treatment. We discussed my starting anti-estrogen, and he phoned in the prescription.

These chemo drugs can cause many problems. I prayed daily for the Lord to protect my heart, liver, and pancreas and for me not to have problems later from the drugs. I also asked him to raise my blood counts. How overwhelming life can be with normal day-to-day stresses joined by complications from medicines that are supposed to make us well!

I was praying to get through the treatments and wishing for better days. I wonder how many people pray to finish their race on earth and have a better day in heaven? Although we should find hope in knowing that day is coming, we need to focus our prayer on what is happening today. In the Lord's Prayer, Jesus said, "Give us this day our daily bread" (Matthew 6:11 ESV).

Today. We must pray about what we feel . . . today. We must be thankful for today and stand firm again evil and temptations . . . today.

And so, each day, we must press onward, trusting God for today. Talking to him about today. Just as we recognize the voice of people we know, he recognizes our voice when we talk to him.

> "The eyes of the Lord watch over those who do right, and his ears are open to their prayers."
>
> — 1 PETER 3:12

Some days we will feel happy, some days drained. But we press onward because God's people will be rewarded in eternal life.

> I press on to reach the end of the race and receive the heavenly prize for which God, through Christ Jesus, is calling us.
>
> — PHILIPPIANS 3:14

Reflections

During a journey like this, it is so easy to let our minds dwell on the what-ifs. The fears. The pain yet to come. The unknown. But we need to remember that God holds the future and has everything under control. No matter what we see happening in the world around us. No matter what is happening in our personal world. No matter what is happening to our body. God is in control. He wants us to be still and trust him.

"Be still, and know that I am God!"

— Psalm 46:10

Stop striving. Stop fearing. Find peace in knowing that he is God. Even when things seem chaotic and confusing to us, He has it all under control.

Jesus said it plainly: "So don't worry about tomorrow, for tomorrow will bring its own worries. Today's trouble is enough for today" (Matthew 6:34).

God has gone before you. Keep your eyes on him.

"Do not be afraid or discouraged, for the Lord will personally go ahead of you. He will be with you; he will neither fail you nor abandon you."

— Deuteronomy 31:8

My Thoughts

76

BE SENSITIVE TO GOD'S PRESENCE

March 11–13, 2022. I was super tired. However, I knew I was not as sick as some taking this treatment and was thankful for that.

Lord, please hold my body in your arms and give me peace and strength. Help me to feel well. Strengthen my bones and body. Lord, clear my mind from fears and concerns. Pick me up and make me strong. Too often I have fear! Satan is trying to steal my joy. Bring me peace and joy.

March 15. David had his second knee replacement and spent the night at the hospital. I went home—too tired to spend the night anywhere else. That day I also began taking the anti-estrogen prescription, which I will be on for five to ten years.

March 16. I was beginning to feel some side effects from the anti-estrogen—more crying and sadness. However, there were some positive things to look forward to. I couldn't wait to play pickleball again. I would also rejoice when the fear and crying subsided. And I was sure David couldn't wait until my cooking got better!

March 17. My brother and his family came to visit and spend a couple of days. Having other people around to help with the laundry and pick up groceries provided more time for me to rest, and I was thankful to have someone to visit with. My prayers continued for healing for both David and me.

Seven more infusions over the next 120 days. With God's help, we can do this! *Lord, thank you for life today. Please protect my heart, liver, and pancreas and raise my blood count. Take away my fear. Sometimes fear of pain or complications overwhelms me. Bring me to the end of this treatment. **It's so hard!** How great thou art, Lord. Give me your power. Praise you, Lord, for your love and strength! Praise you for a husband who loves you and is helping me through this time.*

March 24. My eighth infusion. A friend took me. We ate brunch after; then I went home. After taking the usual Benadryl, I was more than ready to lie down!

Reflections

In the infusion room that day, one of the patients was excitedly talking about finding a cardinal feather on the dash of her car after an accident, and I set out to learn why she was excited. There are a number of legends about the meaning of cardinals—they vary by culture, religion, mythology, and beliefs.

Victoria McGovern wrote a poem claiming, "Cardinals appear when angels are near."[6] Some relate the color of cardinals to the blood of Christ: "The cardinal's red color is a reminder of the blood of Christ. . . . Thus, for some Christians, the spiritual meaning of cardinals relates to the eternal life available through the spilling of Christ's blood."[7]

The cardinal can also be symbolic of combatting difficulties with hope and persistence.[8] This particular symbolism really spoke to me. Later that evening, I was watching birds at my feeder. I could not believe my eyes—there were seven cardinals at the feeder! Including that day, I had seven infusions left. God was using this symbolism to encourage me and fill me with hope! I was even more determined to get through this cancer treatment!

God speaks to different people in various ways. I encourage you to be prayerfully aware of his presence—even in the little things of life. Invite him to fill you with hope!

Through Christ you have come to trust in God. And you have placed your faith and hope in God because he raised Christ from the dead and gave him great glory.

— 1 PETER 1:21

77

DON'T GIVE UP!

April 1–6, 2022. We experienced more fearful days—this time centered around David. He had a high fever and a rash on his legs and generally did not feel well. A visit to the doctor for blood work and X-rays brought back normal results, but he was no better. At first the doctor thought it could be a rejection of the new knee, but it wasn't. Neither was it an infection. The doctor concluded it was a reaction to a drug he was taking. A couple of days after changing his meds, he was feeling well again. By faith, we kept walking!

Amid the up-and-down struggles and fear, the Lord continued helping me. In faith, I kept asking God to heal me. To take away the side effects.

Lord, send your Holy Spirit to surround this house and protect us from Satan's grip and prevent him from stealing my joy.

The joy of the Lord truly was my strength. As I focused on him, Jesus provided me with strength and helped me overcome my fears. The Lord walked with me and helped me remain calm. Friends continued surrounding us with food, cards, and prayers. I hoped that one day we would be able to bless others as we were being blessed.

April 14. My ninth chemo infusion in this last series. Looking back, I reflected on how God had kept us in his hands. Every day is a gift of life. I was thankful for that day and considered how I could make it a happy one. I wanted to make each day count, rejecting self-pity and bitterness. I wanted to put my days of anxiety and fear in the past. The Lord was so much greater than all that.

> Little children, you are from God and have overcome them, for he who is in you is greater than he who is in the world.
>
> — 1 John 4:4 ESV

I knew I must fight to believe in God's power and to overcome. I had heard it said that 75 percent of healing is in the mind, believing God's power. *I believe! I will be healed. I will have energy. I will have no more side effects! God holds me in his hands. His blood has covered me. I will keep loving others and keep pressing onward!*

Reflections

Don't give up! When doubts fill you, ask God to help you believe. "I do believe, but help me overcome my unbelief!" (Mark 9:24).

Are you waiting on the Lord? Keep waiting! He will do all things in his time. Don't trust in circumstances. Don't trust in what you feel. Trust in Jesus and his promises. His ways are perfect, and he is always on time.

The Lord directs our steps, so why try to understand everything along the way?

— PROVERBS 20:24

I long for your blessings, Lord. I think of Job. He suffered, but then you brought him blessings. Lord, you provide breath and give life. I lean on you, Lord. You choose some to go to heaven at a young age and some to have a long life on earth. I do long for no sickness or pain or fear. I long for health, but only you know what will happen.

God is in control. In heaven there will be no more sorrow and no pain. But until that time, it is not wrong to ask for healing. No more sickness or cancer. Don't give up! Trust God to do what is best for you—in his way and his time.

O my people, trust in him at all times. Pour out your heart to him, for God is our refuge.

— Psalm 62:8

78

BECAUSE HE LIVES

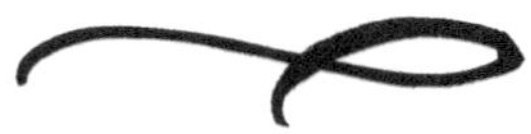

April 17, 2022. Easter Sunday. Although it was very short, I was able to wear my own hair to church. I was thankful a year had passed since my cancer diagnosis, and we were almost through this valley of trials. I was ready to see what God would do at my checkup the following week.

Of course, my thoughts turned to Jesus as we celebrated his resurrection. He gave his life for every person who chooses to believe in him and follow his Word. I think of joy in the morning when I think of Easter. Can you imagine the joy the people experienced when they heard Jesus had risen from the dead? When I was younger, we often had services outside as the sun was coming up. I always felt so much peace and joy thinking of him coming alive, overcoming death. I was rejoicing for the day we will all see Jesus and will have no more pain or sorrow.

A year into my cancer journey, I was alive to celebrate God's gift of salvation. He died so we can have eternal life in heaven—no more sickness!

Looking back at the year, I recorded many blessings. Here are a few:

- Safe trips back and forth from Texas
- No pain from my mastectomy surgery
- Going to my niece's wedding
- Our kids home for Christmas
- Our kids in Texas providing a place for us to live during treatment
- Healing from burns
- My parents remaining well
- David's second knee surgery going so well

I was also thankful for the way friends had blessed us with food, smoothies, gifts, gift cards, money, visits, grocery shopping, cards, books, and so much encouragement. *Oh, Lord, we must count our blessings.*

A song I had sung as a child came to mind. "Count your many blessings, name them one by one; count your blessings, see what God hath done." I could see what God had done during this journey! Blessings upon blessing!

Reflections

If you do not yet know the Lord and how he came to save us, please seek a Christian minister for guidance. And search the Bible. A good place to start is reading the Gospel of John and the book of Romans. Knowing him and experiencing his gift of eternal life is the only way to find true peace.

"For this is how God loved the world: He gave his one and only Son, so that everyone who believes in him will not perish but have eternal life."

— JOHN 3:16

You were dead because of your sins and because your sinful nature was not yet cut away. Then God made you alive with Christ, for he forgave all our sins. He canceled the record of the charges against us and took it away by nailing it to the cross.

— COLOSSIANS 2:13–14

Knowing Jesus personally and learning to trust him will make it possible for you to face all your tomorrows. One song that reminds me of that is "Because He Lives." Because Jesus lives, you can face anything that comes. You don't have to be afraid. Yes, he holds the future for both you and me. And he loves us more than we can imagine.

My Thoughts

79

ONE YEAR LATER

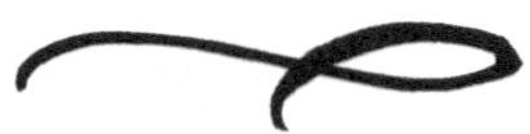

April 25, 2022. It had been a year since this journey began, and we headed to Texas for my one-year checkup. When we had pulled out of our driveway the year before, I had cried and said I may never see my home again. I had so much fear. This time when we pulled out, I said, "I will be back healthy, and we will have good reports."

Sometimes I meet a cancer patient who has experienced only her first few treatments. Often, she asks, "When will this get better?"

I try to explain it is a very hard, fearful journey with ups and downs every day—but it won't last forever. I never had a day without fear, tears, and what-ifs. But I continued refocusing on Jesus. I knew God had forgiven my sins. He took them to the cross. But my enemy, Satan, kept trying to destroy my view of Christ. He messed with me, discouraging me and bringing doubt about Jesus and his love. When I got sick from the chemo, fearful thoughts attacked me, trying to convince me I was losing. *But wait! God is my victory! He will win the battle for me!*

Wherever you are in your cancer journey, I want to encourage you to hold on to God's promises. He will never leave you nor forsake you. He is your strength. Hold on to God's hope! I encourage you to meditate on these Scriptures and others God leads you to.

> The angel of the Lord encamps around those who fear him, and delivers them.
>
> — Psalm 34:7 ESV

> Yet I still belong to you; you hold my right hand. You guide me with your counsel, leading me to a glorious destiny.
>
> — Psalm 73:23–24

> The Lord says, "I will rescue those who love me. I will protect those who trust in my name. When they call on me, I will answer; I will be with them in trouble. I will rescue and honor them. I will reward them with a long life and give them my salvation."
>
> — Psalm 91:14–16

And so, Lord, where do I put my hope? My only hope is in you.

— Psalm 39:7

I know from experience that we drift when we don't stay in God's Word. We will get discouraged if we don't focus on Jesus. But if we do focus on him, he will carry us.

Keep focused. *God, Jesus, life . . . God, Jesus, life . . . God, Jesus, life.*

Reflections

When you are in the midst of pain and suffering, you may feel as if it will go on forever. But God promises joy in the morning!

Weeping may last through the night, but joy comes with the morning.

— Psalm 30:5

Wherever you are in your journey, don't give up! Morning is coming! And with it will come joy!

My Thoughts

80

LORD, MAKE ME SHINE!

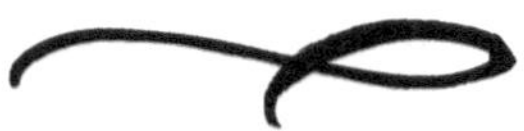

April 26–27, 2022. I had several appointments. The first was with my heart doctor for an ECHO, EKG, aorta scan, and ultrasound of my heart. All were normal! I was so happy that thus far the treatments had not damaged my heart. *Thank you, Lord! Please keep my heart strong to the end.*

Next came the left breast mammogram. Another wonderful report. No signs of any cancer. The place that had been removed during surgery could hardly be seen. My doctor had done a great job. *Thank you, Lord!*

Except for slightly low white blood cell and platelet counts, my labs were normal. Another blessing!

My daughter-in-law Amy went with me to see the oncologist, who was very pleased with all the test reports.

She told me to try to eat more. She said I could increase my exercise a little but not to attempt any big weights or bench presses until I was stronger. She did approve traveling and said I could go to Europe, as planned, after the last chemo. Her words were so encouraging: "You must begin living. Just because you have had cancer, you cannot live as if it were still there. So, begin living and doing whatever you want."

More good news. She said my port could come out a week following my last chemo and scheduled an appointment in August for that to be done in surgery under X-ray.

She cautioned me that breast cancer often returns to the chest wall and to the remaining breast. It can also metastasize to the liver, bone, and colon. The highest rate of recurrence is during the first three years. It's less likely from three to five years and rare after that.

Lord, bring me peace, confidence, and direction for my life. May I be happy and rejoice in you. May I rejoice in all things, as your Word says. I am thankful for the good reports I've just had. I long for health and believe the cancer is gone. I have hope and faith you are walking with me. You are showing your power of healing. You are answering the prayer warriors' petitions for healing. You are rescuing me from this evil cancer!

Reflections

While in Texas, we enjoyed some wonderful family time and went to church a couple of times. Amy and Judy went with me to Nordstrom, where I was fitted for my first prosthesis and bought two bras.

That was so difficult. I struggled not to be fearful or sad. A very hard journey! I had lost part of my body, which had looked good before the breast removal. Now one side was flat, and we worked around the remaining breast. I was so thankful I had chosen to have only one removed and just to monitor the second one. I was happy I didn't have to deal with two protheses—it's hard to keep the one in place, and it's uncomfortable.

One devotional book that had been given to me was about being brave. One of the devotions talks about how pretty a diamond in the rough is when it is shined up. As I followed God through this journey, he had smoothed my rough edges. I was shining brighter and looking forward to the day when I would shine bright like a big diamond! *Lord, keep me from being downcast, and let my soul be at peace. Let me see my value in living and who I am. Please help me move forward with a positive attitude for the future. Lord, may you be shining me up! Smooth my edges so I will be a bright, shining diamond in the years ahead.*

Remember that you are God's special creation. As you walk with him, let that inner beauty shine.

Your adornment must not be merely external—with interweaving and elaborate knotting of the hair, and wearing gold jewelry, or [being superficially preoccupied with] dressing in expensive clothes; but let it be [the inner beauty of] the hidden person of the heart, with the imperishable quality and unfading charm of a gentle and peaceful spirit, [one that is calm and self-controlled, not overanxious, but serene and spiritually mature] which is very precious in the sight of God.

— 1 Peter 3:3–4 AMP

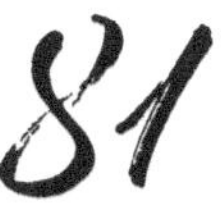

EACH DAY A GIFT

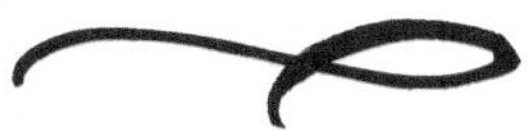

May 5, 2022. Chemo number ten. My blood work was still a little low, but the doctors had assured me it was good, considering all the treatments I'd had. I wasn't as tired as usual after the treatment.

I was looking forward to the beautiful weather that week and planned to get some flowers to plant. Planting them in pots and around the landscaping, I was so blessed to see God's creation blooming. Spring brings me thoughts of the heavens opening and letting the sun shine through to bless us with new life of the trees, shrubs, and grass. I wondered if Jesus will return in the springtime when everything is blooming and birds are singing with happiness. What an unimaginably wonderful and exciting moment that will be when we look up to the heavens and see Jesus coming for those who love him. We must be ready!

May 10–16. David had an infection in his knee and was very sick with a high fever. I was up taking care of him the two nights when his temperature was 104 degrees, and I was tired. Praise God, he gradually recovered.

May 18. I worked on mulch and landscaping and some spring cleaning. I felt super great with the spring cleaning, sparkling windows, and my flowers. I felt alive! I had a more positive attitude and was growing stronger and eating better. However, I did still struggle with bad chemo brain. I don't know how to describe it except to say my brain just wasn't working!

May 26. I had my eleventh chemo treatment. Again, I did better than usual. Although I was still tired, I wasn't crying as much or as depressed. *Lord, give me the strength to press forward for the next three months to the end!*

Reflections

Even the many times I felt tired, I tried to remind myself how special each day was. A gift of life. I appreciated the gift of today, and I knew it was up to me to make each day a happy one. How could I do that? I wanted to be joyful and make *today* count. I determined to resist self-pity and bitterness.

As I neared the end of my treatments, I prayed my days of doubt and an anxious heart were behind me. I knew Jesus had suffered here on earth, but he told us he had overcome, and we can too.

"I have told you all this so that you may have peace in me. Here on earth you will have many trials and sorrows. But take heart, because I have overcome the world."

— JOHN 16:33

I will not fear. I will fight to win this battle and to overcome the things happening to my body. I will believe in God's power.

My doctors said many times that my mind would be 75 percent of my healing. I knew I must have positive thoughts. Positive thoughts of faith. But it was so hard. Why? Because Satan wants to steal our joy. Our confidence in Jesus. And he wants to make us fearful.

Are you experiencing his attacks of fear and doubt? The Bible tells us to resist him and run to God. That's our job. Then God takes care of the rest as we trust him.

Submit yourselves, then, to God. Resist the devil, and he will flee from you. Come near to God and he will come near to you.

— JAMES 4:7–8 NIV

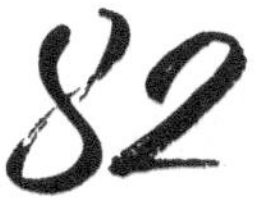

LIVE STRONG

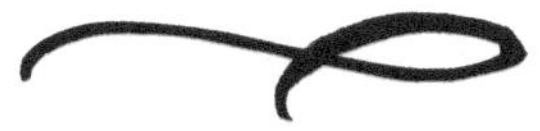

June 2022. A new month.

Lord, keep me stable, calm, confident, peaceful! I thank you for giving me the strength and confidence to get through this treatment. Thank you that I am living! Lord, may I live many more years with health.

My best friend from high school came for the week to have a funeral for her mom and celebrate her life. She had lived to ninety-one, and all her children and grandchildren were still living. What a blessing. She was an example of prayer and how to live through the cancer she had had forty years before. Live strong! Live, love, and believe in God.

Soon the days would pass, and this cancer journey would be behind me. I knew I must be still and know that he is

God. I encourage you to do that too. Rest in Jesus's peace and surrender your feelings of fear. Cancer cannot hold you down—being afraid and yielding to Satan's attack can, though. Walk with Jesus. He is your future.

I know it's not easy to let go of the fear. I could hardly wait to feel great after all the chemo was out of my body. I still feared the what-ifs. Would I be strong and have more years of life? Although I could see improvement, it was difficult to keep hoping and believing I would be better. I had come a long way but was still afraid. I needed God to show me the way.

> Your word is a lamp to guide my feet and a light for my path.
>
> — Psalm 119:105

> I have hidden your word in my heart, that I might not sin against you.
>
> — Psalm 119:11

Reflections

> I continued to trust and hope in the Lord. Some said to me, "Well, it doesn't matter. We all die, and you know where you are going." That's true. But I enjoy life with family and friends, so I was not going to just give up and die.

I believe we must keep our eyes on heaven but not close them to earthly living. We are here for a reason. God wants us to use every opportunity we have to serve and worship him. We cannot just give up living.

Remember Jesus in the garden just before he was arrested and crucified.

Then Jesus went with them to the olive grove called Gethsemane, and he said, "Sit here while I go over there to pray." He took Peter and Zebedee's two sons, James and John, and he became anguished and distressed. He told them, "My soul is crushed with grief to the point of death. Stay here and keep watch with me." He went on a little farther and bowed with his face to the ground, praying, "My Father! If it is possible, let this cup of suffering be taken away from me. Yet I want your will to be done, not mine."

— MATTHEW 26:36–39

Then Jesus left them a second time and prayed, "My Father! If this cup cannot be taken away unless I drink it, your will be done."

— MATTHEW 26:42

So he went to pray a third time, saying the same things again.

— MATTHEW 26:44

Jesus was sorrowful and troubled. Through this cancer journey, I have experienced many times of being sorrowful and troubled—you probably have too. My prayer warriors have carried me through with their prayers for my healing. I continually prayed for the cancer to pass from me.

I knew God was in control. My future was in his hands—his decision. And I trusted him to do what was best. But I also knew I loved my family and enjoyed watching them grow in the Lord. I enjoyed serving and helping others. I knew I was to share this journey with others going through cancer, and I wanted to give them hope to press on and never give up.

As long as you have breath—keep going. Life isn't full of promises, but we are promised that if we follow Jesus, we will have eternal life with him. Press on! Don't give up!

— My Thoughts —

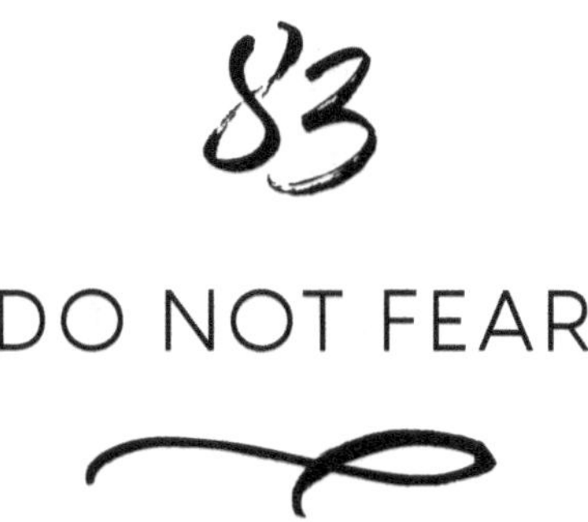

DO NOT FEAR

June 16, 2022. Twelfth chemo infusion. Only two more treatments after this! I couldn't wait to be finished. I wanted to move forward and not think about what to eat or how much to sleep, drink, or exercise. I wanted to be able to just live!

I love you, Lord. I ask for happiness, health, and encouragement to give to others. I know you are the Lord of my life. May Satan be bound and not have control of my health, my mind, or my soul. Bless me with steadfast faith.

God is able to do anything. He can change my whole life!

Not why? Or why me? Yes, Lord, put your arms around me. You have allowed a change in my life, but now you are making another change. You are bringing me healthy days. Your arms are around me, Lord. I feel your healing power and the strength you are providing for me to make it through these last treatments. Only two more to go.

I sat and waited like Job in the Old Testament. He was sick. He had lost his children, land, and animals. But he continued trusting God and was later blessed with much more than he had lost. *Lord, I don't know what blessings you have for me, but I look for your hand to touch me with healing.*

God was in charge. His spirit was around me, and his hands held me up. The touch of the Master's hand!

> "But if you remain in me and my words remain in you, you may ask for anything you want, and it will be granted!"

> — JOHN 15:7

Reflections

During this time, the following Scriptures spoke to me in a special way. I hope they will encourage you as well.

A glad heart makes a happy face; a broken heart crushes the spirit. A wise person is hungry for knowledge, while the fool feeds on trash. For the despondent, every day brings trouble; for the happy heart, life is a continual feast.

> — PROVERBS 15:13–15

O my people, trust in him at all times. Pour out your heart to him, for God is our refuge.

— Psalm 62:8

A cheerful heart is good medicine, but a broken spirit saps a person's strength.

— Proverbs 17:22

"Do not fear" is in the Bible 365 times. The devil tries to control us with fear. He caused me to fear a lot with what-ifs. To combat that, I strived to lean on the Word of God daily. But it was still a daily struggle to refuse to listen to Satan's lies and instead focus on Jesus and his Word. Can you identify with what I'm saying? Fear can pull you down. Hang on to Jesus!

"Don't let your hearts be troubled. Trust in God, and trust also in me."

— John 14:1

Then Jesus said, "Come to me, all of you who are weary and carry heavy burdens, and I will give you rest."

— Matthew 11:28

Let today begin your future. Don't let your past doubts and fears rob you of faith and joy today or affect your hope for the future.

My Thoughts

84

A TIME TO LAUGH

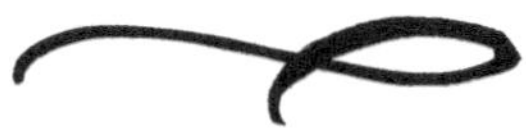

June 19, 2022. Father's Day. Dad and Mom and my brother, Jeff, and his family joined us for lunch. The house was full of laughter and family. This special time together brought me life and hope and encouragement to keep pressing on. I was delighted that Jeff and his family were able to stay several days.

July 4. We spent the day with Mom and Dad.

July 7. This should have been the day for my thirteenth infusion, but they had forgotten to order my meds. Perhaps the holiday interfered, but I was upset about the delay. If too much time elapsed, I would need an extra booster dose. But that didn't happen. I had number thirteen on July 12, and my last treatment was moved ahead to August 2.

I wanted these treatments behind me and prayed daily I could finish. My chemo brain was making it hard to stay focused. My mind could not handle more than one thought at a time. When someone asked me a question, my mind took a while to process it. I was praying for my brain cells to regrow quickly after the final chemo.

July 13. David's birthday. *Lord, bless David for his steadfast encouragement for me as I pressed through the cancer treatments. Thank you for your continued provision when I hurt and fear, when I feel sad.*

July 19. *Lord, please bless us with happy days and health for our family. Bless us with faithful children. Lord, you have held me through the difficult days. I believe you touched me and took all cancer away from me forever!*

I am almost done. I will move forward!

> Take delight in the Lord, and he will give you your heart's desires.
>
> — Psalm 37:4

> Let us seize and hold tightly the confession of our hope without wavering, for He who promised is reliable and trustworthy and faithful [to His word].
>
> — Hebrews 10:23 AMP

Reflections

That week of family time meant so much to me. The laughter. The sharing. It helped me focus less on what was yet to come and the what-ifs—and more on the love that surrounded me. I was able to relax and enjoy myself.

When you are feeling especially low . . . or fearful . . . or frustrated about things like rescheduled appointments, I encourage you to spend some time with people you care about. Play games. Take a drive. Invite them over to just "hang out." Laugh about fun memories. What a difference it can make!

For everything there is a season, a time for every activity under heaven. . . . A time to cry and a time to laugh. A time to grieve and a time to dance.

— ECCLESIASTES 3:1, 4

Take time to laugh and dance!

— My Thoughts —

85

ALL THINGS

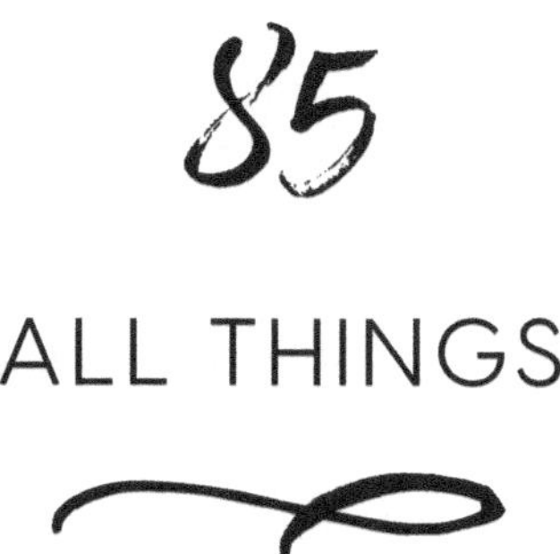

July 20, 2022. I was feeling discouraged and fearful again. Weakness limited what I could do. I was sad thinking of all I had done in the past that I had not been able to do through this cancer journey. I was just sitting, not doing much to help us—or anyone else. Do you ever feel like that?

Lord, please help me do for others and show appreciation to my team of caregivers for all they've done. I want to celebrate the last treatment—with them!

I must keep my eyes on Jesus.

Lord, I don't like being weak and sick. Please give me strength. Will I be in heaven someday? Will I live beyond these seventy years? Lord, keep your hand on me.

July 26. Twenty-three days left for one more chemo treatment, having an ECHO, and my port coming out! After that I would not have weekly appointments and tests. I would not be taking those chemo drugs. I would slowly get back to normal and feel like myself.

Lord, during these past 475 days of sickness and weakness, you have kept your arms around me. You have held me through the nights of sickness, sadness, and fear. Lord, I am grateful to you for the strength you have given me.

Lord, may I be well again. May I live the days of my life ahead in health. I know you are the great provider. You hold everything in your hands. Praise you, Lord! I am grateful to know you and your Word.

May I be blessed to be in your presence at the end of my life on earth. I ask for more days to enjoy with my family. Lord, protect my family from the evil one.

Praise you, Lord. Praise your holy name! May there be joy in the days ahead.

Although heaven is in my future someday, I would have joy in the Lord even while still on earth. *Today is the day of the Lord!*

My last chemo was fast approaching. Celebration to come!

Reflections

I would be returning to Texas for my port to be removed. Seven years before, I had not been thrilled when Chris and his family moved to Texas. But now, even in that, I could see God at work. Now I was so thankful they had moved to Houston. Because of that, we were able to stay with them while I had cancer treatments at the best cancer treatment center in the world (in my opinion).

How many other things that I didn't understand at the time has God used for good? Countless, I am sure. And I believe with all my heart, he is bringing good even from my cancer surgery—only time will tell what all those good things will be.

You, like me, have probably wondered many times through your cancer journey what possible good could come from it. Even when we can't see any possibility of good, we need to remember that God promised he will bring good from *all* things to those who love him.

And we know [with great confidence] that God [who is deeply concerned about us] causes all things to work together [as a plan] for good for those who love God, to those who are called according to His plan and purpose.

— ROMANS 8:28 AMP

My Thoughts

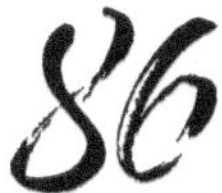

RING THE BELL!

August 2, 2022. My fourteenth chemo treatment in the second series. The last one! My cancer treatment was almost behind me—that was reason for a great celebration. I was so excited and could hardly believe I had made it to the final day of the journey.

It was a wonderful opportunity to show my appreciation to the medical teams in Joplin who had helped me so much. I gave the doctor and the two primary infusion nurses special gifts. I also made two large candy bar bouquets so every staff member could have one. To that I added a basket of small candy bars to offer variety.

Amid all the excitement and emotions, I knew I had to stay focused to get through the infusion. As I finished the process, I felt tired and weak, as usual. But I was filled with joy as I stepped into the lobby to ring that bell of celebration.

Space was limited, but I had invited as many as possible of my prayer warriors to join me. Some of them couldn't come because of work, and some lived too far away.

The invitation I sent began this way:

Celebration Invitation to Bell Ringing
following my **final chemo infusion**

Tuesday, August 2, 2022!!!

I followed that with the details and an additional invitation to be my guest at Cracker Barrel for brunch to continue the celebration. I also included a note of thanks for all they had done. "Please stand beside me that day and represent the many hundreds around the world who have lifted me up in prayer for strength and healing."

This was the moment. Infusion completed, I stepped into the lobby to a room filled with forty-two friends. They all clapped and praised the Lord with me. First, I rang a personal bell I had received from my high school best friend. Then I rang the hospital's bell. I rang and rang!

I had fought. I had endured. And now I rang the bell in celebration.

Praise your name, Lord! I will live until you take my last breath. I pray for health from this day forward!

Reflections

God had allowed the treatments to kill all the cancer. He could have removed it without any treatments, but he had chosen for me to walk this journey. Although I often experienced discouragement and fear, and sometimes my faith wavered, God had provided me strength for the journey!

Someday I will live eternal life in heaven because Jesus saved me by paying the debt for my sins when he died on the cross. The cross in my tree still reminds me of his love. Jesus walked through his journey to the cross, suffered torture, and then died—for me, and for you.

You may still be walking through the pain, suffering, fears, and doubt. I urge you to keep your eyes on Jesus. Don't give up! God will provide strength for your journey, just as he did for me. Take one day at a time. No matter what comes, Jesus is with you.

God is your refuge, your help in trouble. He has already won the battle for you. Greater is he that is in you than he that is in the world. May he hold you steadfast with peace and rest.

Fight to recover! Don't let stress or sadness depress your immune system. Know that God is for you, and you have a reason to live. Cling to him.

God is our refuge and strength, always ready to help in times of trouble. So we will not fear when earthquakes come and the mountains crumble into the sea. Let the oceans roar and foam. Let the mountains tremble as the waters surge!

— Psalm 46:1–3

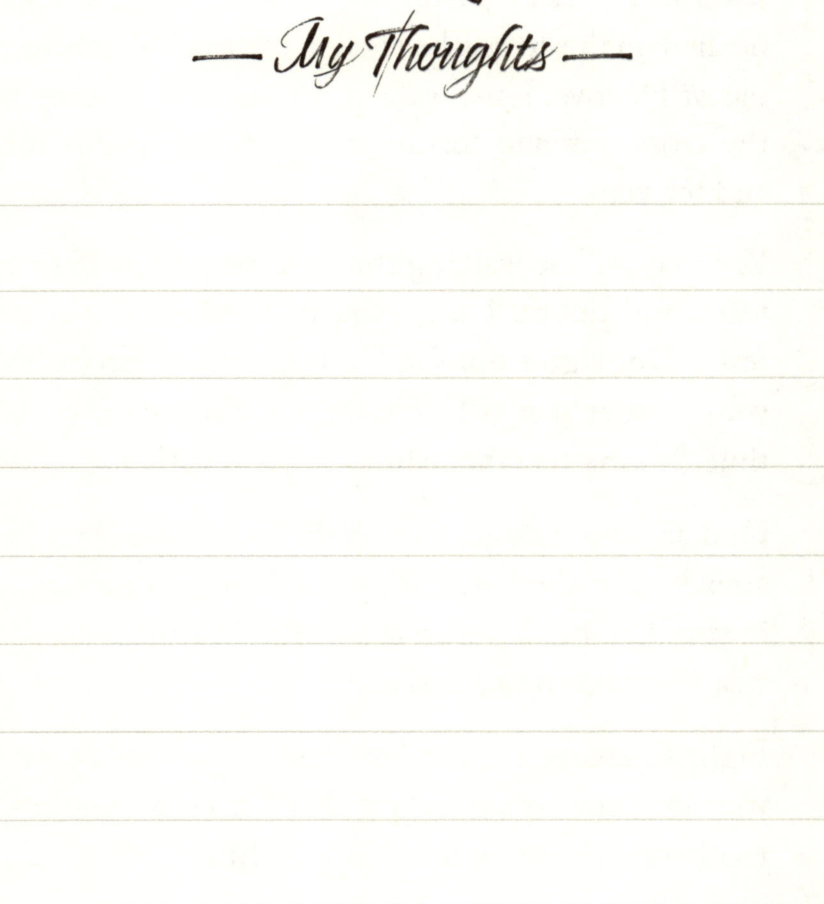

358

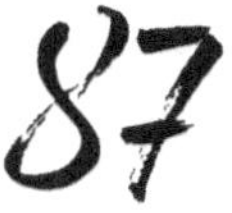

CANCER REMISSION

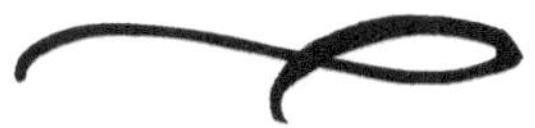

August 15–16, 2022. I returned to MD Anderson mid-August to have my infusion port removed after the final blood work and heart tests.

August 17–18. I had an ECHO, EKG, aorta scan, and ultrasound of my heart. After the tests, my heart doctor said, "Congratulations! You made it through the treatments. Your heart has no damage from the drugs. It is strong. You do have slightly more valve leakage than when we began, but it isn't bad. We will watch it."

My oncologist said I was in remission as of that day! After five years with no recurrence, I would be a survivor of cancer. I would be taking the anti-estrogen medicine for five years. She predicted only a 5 percent chance of the cancer returning. That meant a 95 percent chance it would not! She continued, "When you came to me your first visit, you were my healthiest and most socially active over-seventy patient I ever had. Now after chemo and all the treatments, you are the healthiest, most socially active patient I have ever had. You have done well through this journey." She encouraged me to eat better and build up more strength. Most importantly, she encouraged me to move forward and enjoy my life!

Praise the Lord!

Following the meeting with my doctor, I went to the surgery area, where they removed the port in my left shoulder. I was awake and talking during the procedure.

I would move forward healing and rebuilding my strength for visiting with friends, traveling, working out at the Y, playing pickleball, and bowling. It would be a gradual process, but it was happening!

Reflections

Lord, this journey has been difficult and filled with fear. Please continue providing me with strength through your mercy, power, and love. I am sorry for the fear and doubt. I believe the evil one wants to bring me down, but the power of your healing hands is much more powerful than Satan's schemes. You have heaven waiting for us. A place where no more sickness or fears or trials from Satan can come. Lord, please surround us with your angels and your Holy Spirit to bring us peace and protection.

Lord, I rejoice in your name and thank you for your power, strength, and love. Weakness came, but you provided me with strength. Fear attacked, but you provided me with peace. Sickness invaded my body, but you provided me with healing.

As you walk through your journey, I again encourage you to stay in God's Word. I received so much strength through Scripture. The story of Noah and the flood reminded me how God had cared for him through his journey. When he boarded the ark, he did not know what would happen. He had never seen rain or a flood. He didn't know how long the journey would last or what would happen. But he remained faithful, and God brought him through.

You don't know what will happen through your journey. You don't know how long it will last. But as you trust God, you can know that he will be with you. Nothing can separate you from his love.

Can anything ever separate us from Christ's love? Does it mean he no longer loves us if we have trouble or calamity, or are persecuted, or hungry, or destitute, or in danger, or threatened with death? (As the Scriptures say, "For your sake we are killed every day; we are being slaughtered like sheep.") No, despite all these things, overwhelming victory is ours through Christ, who loved us. And I am convinced that nothing can ever separate us from God's love. Neither death nor life, neither angels nor demons, neither our fears for today nor our worries about tomorrow—not even the powers of hell can separate us from God's love. No power in the sky above or in the earth below—indeed, nothing in all creation will ever be able to separate us from the love of God that is revealed in Christ Jesus our Lord.

— ROMANS 8:35–39

— *My Thoughts* —

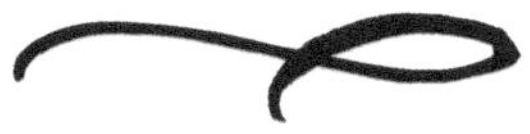

MORE RAINBOWS

The removal of the port ended another phase of my cancer journey. That evening, my son and I sat in the garage watching it rain and thinking God may send another rainbow. Remember my first one? A double rainbow outside Chris's home the night before my first chemo treatment. I believe God was telling me, "Hold on for this boat ride. It will be hard and long, but I am here with the promise to keep you safe." I held on to that promise but often wondered where the boat would land and when the rains and floods would stop. I felt I was drowning with each test, biopsy, treatment, and surgery.

Then there was the second rainbow—over our house this time—the day we returned home after my surgery. I believed the storm was ending, and God was reminding me he is in charge. Then I began more chemo and radiation. I waited daily for the Lord to stop the storm. Now, finally, the storm was ending. *Thank you, God, for holding me through the storm!*

As Chris and I sat there, hoping to see another rainbow, we talked of God's faithfulness throughout this journey. But this day the weather was overcast, and we didn't see a rainbow. In fact, the rain continued for three days.

David and I left in the rain on Monday to head home. In Dallas, some roads were closed because of flooding. Then my phone rang. It was Chris. "Mom, you left too soon! It has just stopped raining, and over our backyard, there is a rainbow!" He sent pictures.

I think this rainbow was for me. Another major part of my treatment was finished after eighteen months.

The first rainbow had been a sign of God's promise to Noah he would never again destroy the earth with a flood. A promise of mercy. And God continued to show me so much mercy.

There was one more rainbow to come. On September 11, we left for Germany on a Danube River cruise. This trip had been planned two years before to celebrate our fiftieth anniversary but had been delayed because of COVID. On the final day of the trip, we were touring Budapest, and another message from God appeared—a huge rainbow over the largest parliament building. It was perfect and reached all the way to the ground. Another message from God. He had seen me through the journey . . . and here I was, moving forward with my life.

Reflections

God is with you as well. Protecting you. Guiding you. Helping you. Encouraging you. He may not encourage you with a cross in a tree or with rainbows, but he will encourage you in ways he knows will bless *you*. Encouragement designed for you alone.

Let me leave you with a Bible event that gave me so much strength through the journey. It is found in Matthew 14:22–31. The disciples were in a boat being battered by a storm. Then they saw Jesus walking on the water toward them. Peter asked Jesus to enable him to walk on the water toward him. Jesus said, "Yes, come." Peter jumped out of the boat and began walking toward Jesus, gazing at him. But then the disciple's eyes strayed to the stormy waves, and he began to sink. He was fine as long as he was focusing on Jesus, but when he refocused on the storm, he began to sink. Even then, when he cried out to Jesus, the Lord reached out and grabbed him, bringing him to safety.

Keep your focus on Jesus. When your attention is taken over by the storm and fear begins to overtake you, call out to Jesus. He will reach out and grab you—and bring you to safety. Nothing can separate you from his love.

Search for the Lord and for his strength; continually seek him.

— Psalm 105:4

♡
— *My Thoughts* —

EPILOGUE

August 2023. I am celebrating a year of remission this August. I'd like to give you an overview of how things have been going during that year.

The first month I was able to travel to Germany to see the passion play in Oberammergau and went on a Danube River cruise. Although I was still not eating well and often taking an afternoon nap, I did very well keeping up with the tours—even with all the walking!

The first six months after treatments were still difficult. Some days I was super tired and weak. Off and on diarrhea continued to be part of my life. For months, mood swings came with crying and fear of a relapse. I found I still had chemo brain, but all my side effects were improving.

My hair has grown faster and needs shaping more regularly. It is so different. Before chemo it was thin, straight, and blond. Now it is thick, curly, and gray. I love my new hair! This wonderful change reminds me who is in control of my healing. Only God could have given me this hair!

Over the months, my mastectomy arm has grown stronger, with good range of motion. Over the first eight months, I still often had lymphedema under the armpit.

Massage therapy helped by moving the fluid to other lymph nodes. My arm is now strong enough for lifting weights up to fifteen pounds (before cancer I had lifted thirty to forty pounds, three times a week). The incision area is less tender, allowing me to wear a prothesis all day long most days.

I have continued increasing my exercising each week, occasionally taking a day or two off for rest and recovery. I am making progress, although it will be some time before I am exercising at the levels I did before my cancer journey. I returned to playing pickleball four months after my last chemo, beginning slowly, with one or two games twice a week. Now I am able to play four or five games three or four days a week (almost back to normal). I continue to walk two or three miles several times each week. (My goal is to return to my previous four miles three to four times a week.) I hope to return to bowling in the fall.

I returned to MD Anderson Cancer Center in April 2023 (the second anniversary of my diagnosis) for a checkup. I had a mammogram and ultrasound of the remaining breast and also saw my heart doctor. After the EKG and echocardiogram of my heart, the cardiologist excitedly told me my heart valve had less leakage, and my heart had gotten stronger. My blood work was all in normal range! I have no permanent damage from the chemo drugs. I rejoiced and praised the Lord as each cancer test came back negative.

After about six months, I began noticing I was not having as much brain fog. I could remember what I needed when I went to the store and was beginning to have longer conversations without forgetting what I wanted to say or what we were talking about.

I still have some neuropathy in my toes and fingertips, but that is improving each month. My nails have begun growing and are not breaking off in the quick any longer. They are now strong enough to scratch my head without bending backward and breaking off.

Sadness, fear, and crying no longer invade my days. Happiness is replacing them. I am able to encourage other cancer patients to hang on and press forward. Also, I am able to share my story more easily without crying—even when I tell someone about the side effects I had or about my fears.

The chemo drugs can cause blurred vision, watery eyes, and eye damage, so I was advised not to change my eyeglass prescription during treatment. The eyes need time to heal after chemo and may get better after about six months. When I went for an exam eight months after my final chemo, the doctor first took my medical history and the list of chemo drugs I had been given. Looking up, she said, "Two of these drugs are the worst drugs for the eyes, so tell me how your eyes are."

I began telling her I had been able to drive since my third chemo treatment with slightly blurry vision in my left eye at a distance. She was very surprised I had been able to drive during the treatment. Then she took a look into my eyes. Quickly she said, "Oh, my!" My heart sank, and fear rushed through my veins.

She continued, "These are the healthiest eyes I've ever seen after chemo, and especially for someone over seventy!" (There they go again talking about my being old!) "You have a very small cataract on both eyes. They are very new and are from the chemo. I don't expect them to get any worse since you have completed the chemo drugs. Also, your vision hasn't changed since your last prescription four years ago!"

I began to cry and praise the Lord. "Only God could have done this. I have been blessed."

I had asked God to protect my eyes over the months of treatment. I had asked him to provide his hand of protection so no organ would get damaged from the chemo drugs. I had hoped in the Lord . . . and was so excited to see how he answered my prayers. My heart, my blood work, and now my eyes. Again, he had demonstrated his power of protection.

So be strong and courageous, all you who put your hope in the Lord!

— PSALM 31:24

But if we look forward to something we don't yet have, we must wait patiently and confidently.

— ROMANS 8:25

One of my prayer requests through my treatment was that I could see my grandchildren graduate. I recently watched my oldest grandchild walk across the stage for his high school graduation in North Carolina! Another wonderful answer to prayer.

A few weeks later, our sons (from North Carolina and Texas), along with their families, met us in Gulf Shores to celebrate. And celebrate we did! Our fifty-third anniversary, our grandson's graduation, and my one-year remission! I enjoyed every day with laughs, food, and time at the beach. We built sandcastles, found seashells, and swam in the pool. Another gift from God.

Overall, I am doing very well! I am so grateful for the days and months I have been blessed to live. God brings me strength and hope on the days I become tired or fear begins.

Many times over these years of treatment and remission, God has carried me. At those times there was only one set of footprints in the sand because God held me in his arms. Now there are two sets walking side by side. God is walking with me every day!

Life has many challenges because Satan is walking around to see who he can devour. He will steal and kill anyone he can. We need to stand firm and, when we have stood a while, continue to stand firm.

And God's promise in Romans 8:28 that God works all things together for good for those who love him? During the painful journey, that can be hard to believe. But he does! I am seeing more evidence of that every day as people diagnosed with cancer call me. God is opening so many doors for me to comfort others the way he comforted me.

> All praise to God, the Father of our Lord Jesus Christ. God is our merciful Father and the source of all comfort. He comforts us in all our troubles so that we can comfort others. When they are troubled, we will be able to give them the same comfort God has given us.
>
> — 2 Corinthians 1:3–4

Recently a friend said to me, "Vicki, you seem more like your old self!"

I laughed. "What does that mean?"

"You laugh a lot like you used to. Your face shines—you are glowing with happiness. You don't have a downcast look in your eyes or facial expressions. Your color is no longer gray, and your eyes sparkle. You act as if you can tackle the day with a peppy attitude."

Yes, God brought me through the darkness back into the light. He has continued to walk beside me and hold me up through the healing and post chemo. I press forward for the five years of remission . . . and then to continue living cancer-free.

Whatever darkness you may be experiencing—whether it's breast cancer or any other kind of heartache and pain—I hope you will trust the Lord to carry you through it. God is there with you. Seek the Lord with your whole heart. He will walk with you through the valley.

A handwritten note from my mom at the time of my diagnosis stands on a small easel in my kitchen:

> Don't you know that day dawns after night, showers displace drought, and spring and summer follow winter? Then, have hope! Hope forever for God will not fail you!

— CHARLES SPURGEON[9]

May you find hope in Jesus.

VICKI'S JOURNEY

By Linda Starkweather, a friend

Vicki arose one morning,
Looked out the window
And what did she see?
It looked like a cross carved in the tree.

David went outside
To see what he could see.
And sure enough,
There was a cross on their tree.

As Vicki looked at that cross,
Day after day,
She remembered how much God loved her,
And the price he had to pay.

Little did she know
That just around the bend,
She would walk a path of suffering
That she often felt would never end.

She began to journal
Her feelings and thoughts!
Even her anger at God
That she had to walk this walk.

But she turned to God's Word,
And his comfort she found.
Trusting her Savior
Through all the ups and downs.

When her body and faith
Grew so very weak
She leaned on family and friends,
Their prayers to seek.

Vicki struggled and strived
With each chemo round
To show God's grace
To those all around.

She began to pass out bracelets
To those who helped her along the way.
It was her way to say thank you,
Love you, and please remember to pray.

As Vicki's boat of faith rocked over the waves,
She began to wonder if God was still there.
So God sent a rainbow on four separate days.
Oh, I promise, my child,
I'm here and I care!

She rang the bell
On August the Second of 2022.
She was so thankful
That her treatments were through!

What comes next only God knows,
Since into the future she cannot look.
She will wait to see. Who knows?
Maybe—she will write a book.

SONGS OF ENCOURAGEMENT

Here are some of the songs that brought me strength during the battle. I hope listening to and singing these and others you know will bring you peace and strength as they draw your focus to Jesus.

"Because He Lives"

"Count Your Blessings"

"Defender"

"Do It Again"

"Fear Is a Liar"

"God Is So Good"

"God on the Mountain"

"God, Turn It Around"

"Got Any Rivers"

"He Touched Me"

"How Great Thou Art"

"I Know"

"I Will Rescue You"

"In Jesus' Name"

"In the Garden"

"Out of My Hands"

"You Alone"

"You've Never Failed Me Yet"

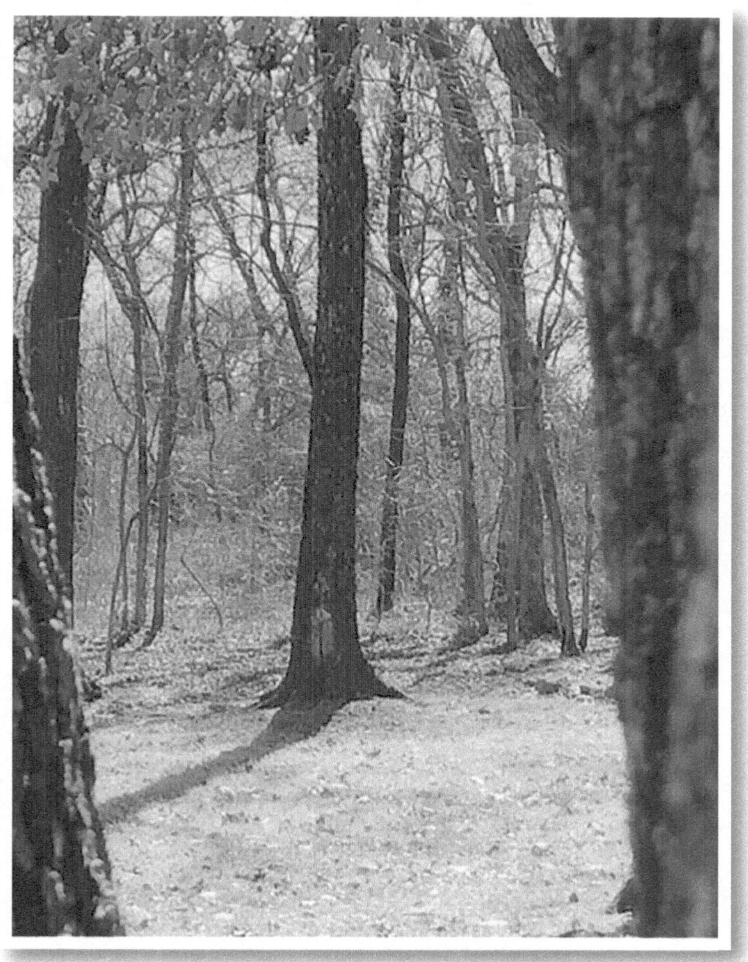

Cross in the tree

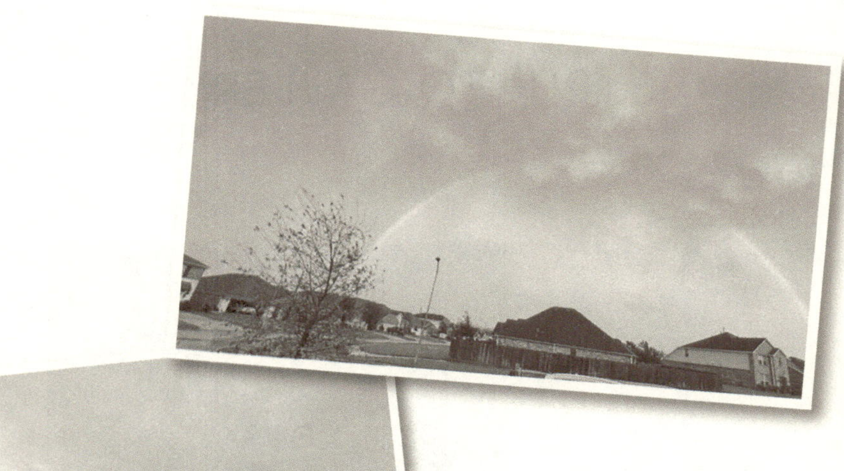

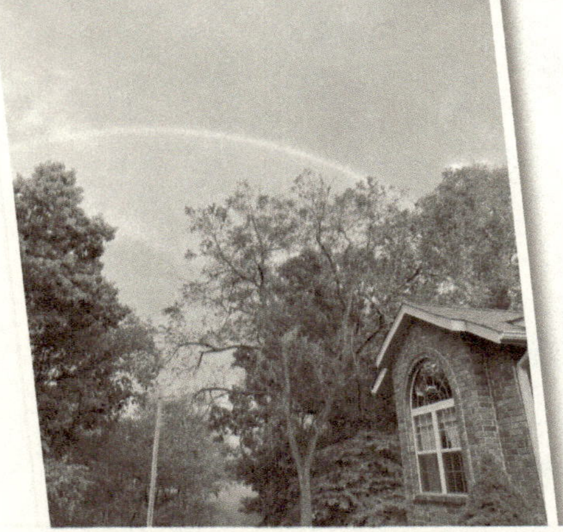

Top: First rainbow

Middle: Arriving home following first six months of chemo and surgery in Texas

Bottom: Last rainbow after final treatments and removal of infusion port . . . Budapest, September 18, 2022

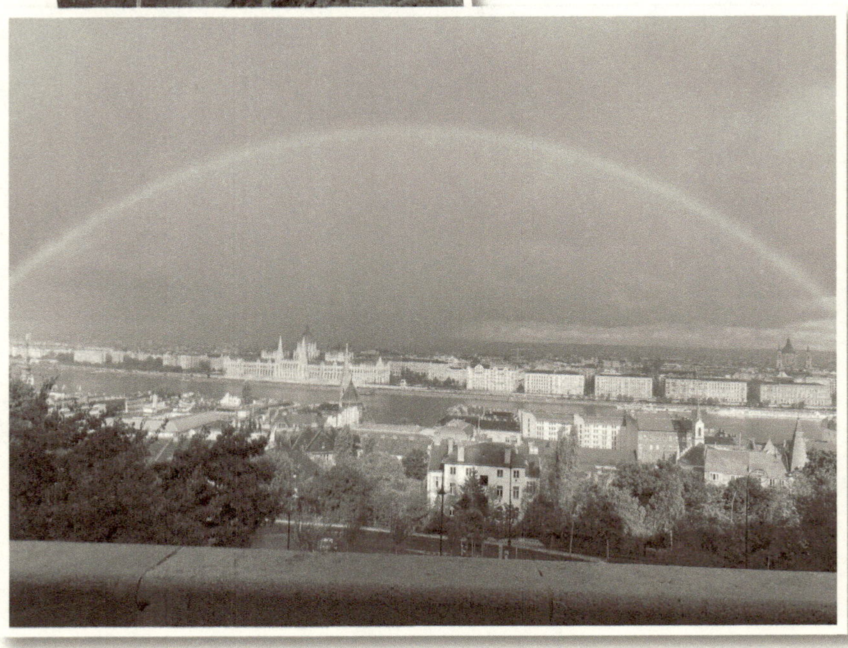

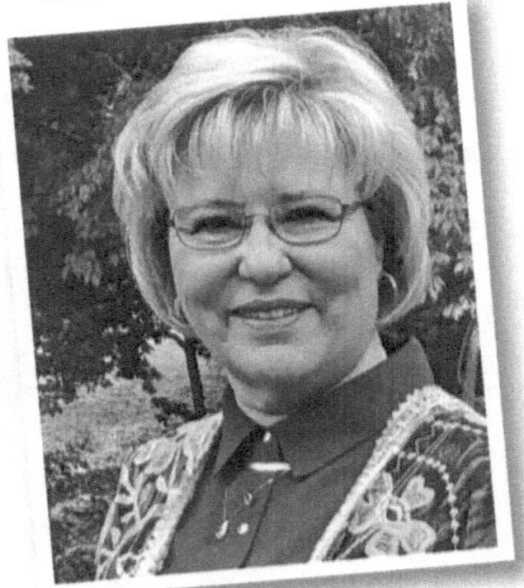

Before cancer journey

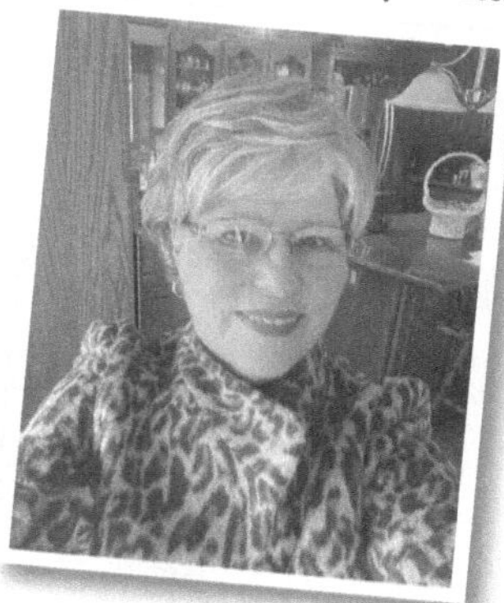

Middle of treatment (my favorite wig)

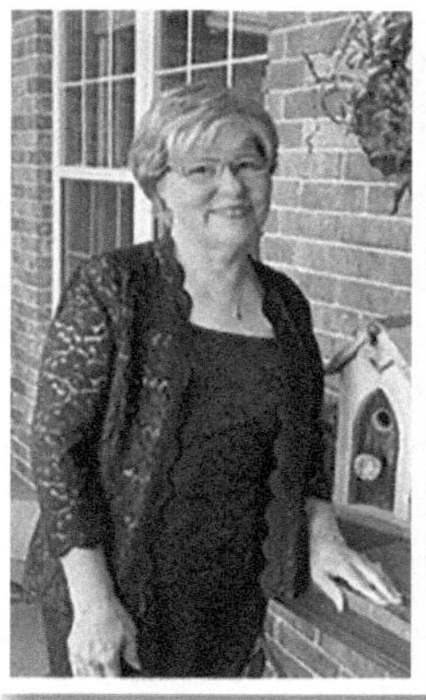

Dressed for niece's wedding
two weeks after surgery

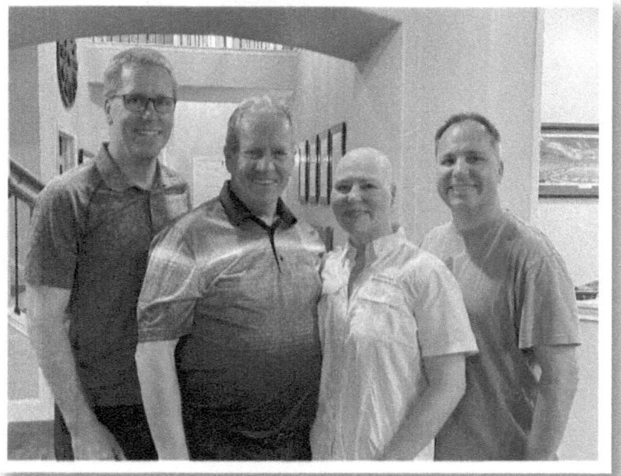

The day they shaved my head

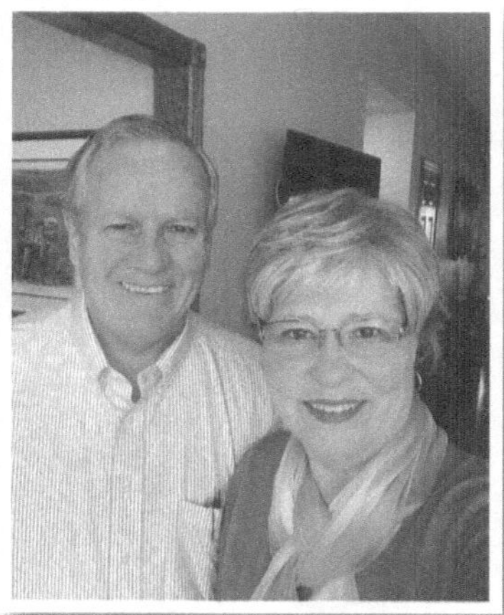

During treatment—great wig

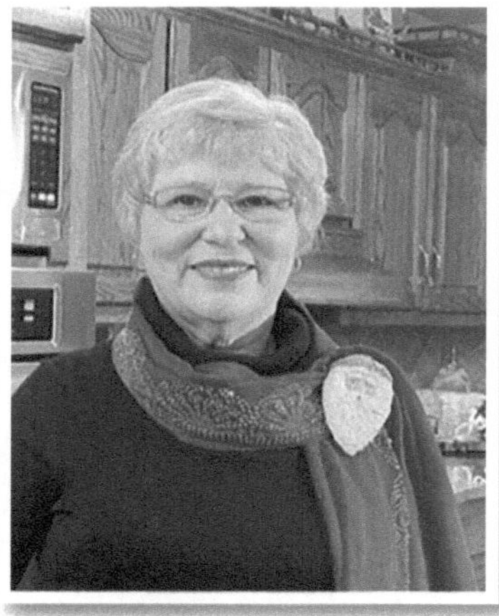

Four months after all
treatments finished

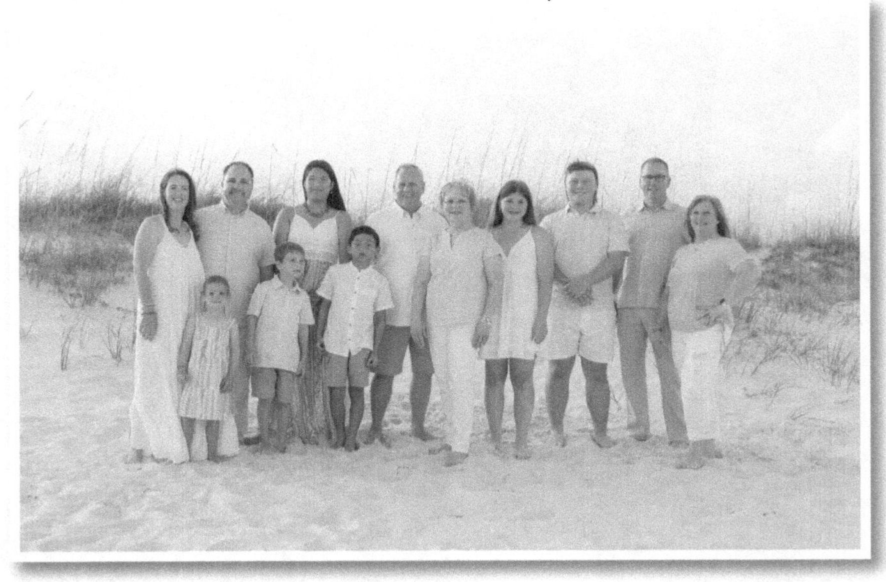

From left: Amy, Chris, Ava, David, Vicki, Larkin, Sheldon, Shon, Michelle
Front row young children: Cora, Sawyer, Silas

Gulf Shores celebration with family one year after treatment

Vicki and David

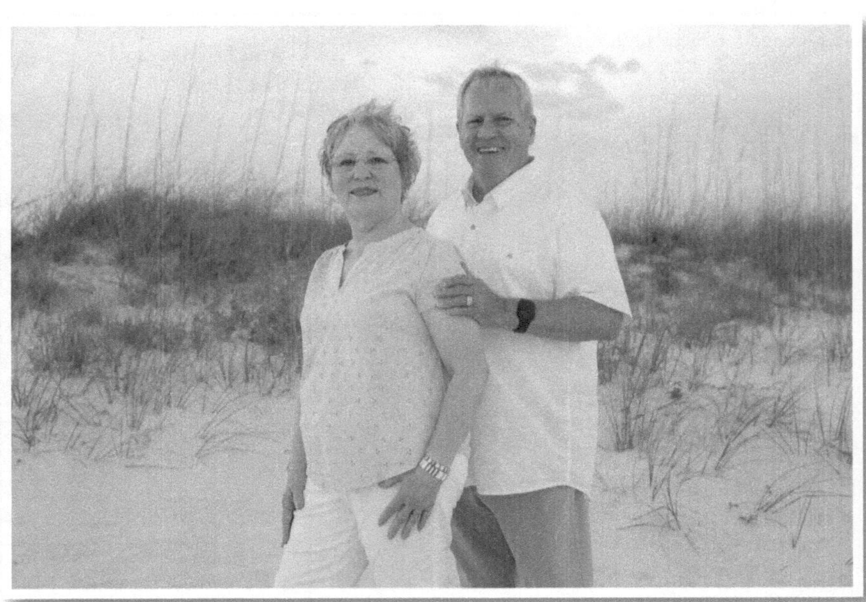

ENDNOTES

1   *Merriam-Webster*, s.v. "hope (*v.*)," accessed August 6, 2023, https://www.merriam-webster.com/dictionary/hope.

2   *Merriam-Webster*, s.v. "trust (*n.*)," accessed August 6, 2023, https://www.merriam-webster.com/dictionary/trust.

3   Charles Spurgeon, quoted in L. B. Cowman, "September 25," in *Streams in the Desert: 366 Daily Devotional Readings*, ed. Jim Reimann (Grand Rapids, MI: Zondervan, 1997), 358.

4   Joyce Meyer, *The Power of Simple Prayer: How to Talk with God about Everything* (New York: FaithWords, 2007), viii, 64–65. Quoted in "Powerful Prayer," *One Passion One Devotion* (blog), published April 18, 2012, https://onepassiononedevotion. wordpress.com/2012/04/18/powerful-prayer/.

5   "Make Your Health Journey Easier with CaringBridge," How It Works, CaringBridge, accessed August 7, 2023, https://www. caringbridge.org/how-it-works/.

6   Amy Wolkenhauer, "15 Famous Poems About Cardinals for a Funeral or Memorial," *Cake* (blog), last updated May 28, 2022, https://www.joincake.com/blog/poems-about-cardinals-and-death/.

7   Tammy Poppie, "Cardinal Meaning & Symbolism: The Ultimate Guide," On the Feeder, published February 24, 2023, https://www.onthefeeder.com/cardinal-meaning-symbolism/.

8   Tom May, "Exploring Red Cardinal Biblical Meaning and Symbolism," Love to Know, published October 14, 2020, https://www.lovetoknow.com/life/grief-loss/exploring-red-cardinal-biblical-meaning-symbolism.

9   Charles Spurgeon, quoted in L. B. Cowman, "September 25," in *Streams in the Desert: 366 Daily Devotional Readings*, ed. Jim Reimann (Grand Rapids, MI: Zondervan, 1997), 358.

SCRIPTURE INDEX

And God said, "This is the sign of the covenant I am making between me and you and every living creature with you, a covenant for all generations to come: I have set my rainbow in the clouds, and it will be the sign of the covenant between me and the earth. Whenever I bring clouds over the earth and the rainbow appears in the clouds, I will remember my covenant between me and you and all living creatures of every kind. Never again will the waters become a flood to destroy all life. Whenever the rainbow appears in the clouds, I will see it and remember the everlasting covenant between God and all living creatures of every kind on the earth."

Genesis 9:12–16 NIV

Chapters 29, 58 (vv. 14–16)

"What's more, I am with you, and I will protect you wherever you go. One day I will bring you back to this land. I will not leave you until I have finished giving you everything I have promised you."

Genesis 28:15

Chapter 67

"The Lord himself will fight for you. Just stay calm."

Exodus 14:14

Chapter 71

"So be strong and courageous! Do not be afraid and do not panic before them. For the Lord your God will personally go ahead of you. He will neither fail you nor abandon you."

Deuteronomy 31:6

Chapter 12

"Do not be afraid or discouraged, for the LORD will personally go ahead of you. He will be with you; he will neither fail you nor abandon you."
Deuteronomy 31:8
Chapters 11, 67, 75

"This is my command—be strong and courageous! Do not be afraid or discouraged. For the LORD your God is with you wherever you go."
Joshua 1:9
Chapters 42, 50

"You come to me with sword, spear, and javelin, but I come to you in the name of the LORD of Heaven's Armies—the God of the armies of Israel, whom you have defied. Today the LORD will conquer you, and I will kill you and cut off your head. And then I will give the dead bodies of your men to the birds and wild animals, and the whole world will know that there is a God in Israel!"
1 Samuel 17:45–46
Chapter 34

"The joy of the LORD is your strength!"
Nehemiah 8:10
Chapter 73

Having hope will give you courage. You will be protected and will rest in safety.
Job 11:18
Chapter 66

The Lord is a shelter for the oppressed, a refuge in times of trouble. Those who know your name trust in you, for you, O Lord, do not abandon those who search for you.

Psalm 9:9–10

Chapter 54

I know the Lord is always with me. I will not be shaken, for he is right beside me.

Psalm 16:8

Chapter 59

The Lord is my shepherd; I have all that I need. He lets me rest in green meadows; he leads me beside peaceful streams. He renews my strength. He guides me along right paths, bringing honor to his name. Even when I walk through the darkest valley, I will not be afraid, for you are close beside me. Your rod and your staff protect and comfort me. You prepare a feast for me in the presence of my enemies. You honor me by anointing my head with oil. My cup overflows with blessings. Surely your goodness and unfailing love will pursue me all the days of my life, and I will live in the house of the Lord forever.

Psalm 23

Chapter 71

Even when I walk through the darkest valley, *I will not be afraid*, for you are close beside me. Your rod and your staff protect and comfort me.

Psalm 23:4 (emphasis mine)

Chapter 35

Yet I am confident I will see the Lord's goodness while I am here in the land of the living.

Psalm 27:13

Chapter 65

Wait for the Lord; be strong and take heart and wait for the Lord.

Psalm 27:14 NIV

Chapter 24

Weeping may last through the night, but joy comes with the morning.

Psalm 30:5

Chapter 79

So be strong and courageous, all you who put your hope in the Lord!

Psalm 31:24

Chapter 66

Epilogue

Unfailing love surrounds those who trust the Lord.

Psalm 32:10

Chapter 74

I prayed to the Lord, and he answered me. He freed me from all my fears.

Psalm 34:4

Chapter 69

The angel of the Lᴏʀᴅ encamps around those who fear him, and delivers them.

Psalm 34:7 ESV

Chapter 79

The Lᴏʀᴅ hears his people when they call to him for help. He rescues them from all their troubles. The Lᴏʀᴅ is close to the brokenhearted; he rescues those whose spirits are crushed.

Psalm 34:17–18

Chapter 25

Take delight in the Lᴏʀᴅ, and he will give you your heart's desires.

Psalm 37:4

Chapter 84

The Lᴏʀᴅ directs the steps of the godly. He delights in every detail of their lives. Though they stumble, they will never fall, for the Lᴏʀᴅ holds them by the hand.

Psalm 37:23–24

Chapter 59

Lᴏʀᴅ, I wait for you; you will answer, Lord my God.

Psalm 38:15 NIV

Chapter 2

And so, Lord, where do I put my hope? My only hope is in you.

Psalm 39:7

Chapters 1, 47, 79

But each day the LORD pours his unfailing love upon me, and through each night I sing his songs, praying to God who gives me life.

Psalm 42:8

Chapter 35

God is our refuge and strength, always ready to help in times of trouble. So we will not fear when earthquakes come and the mountains crumble into the sea. Let the oceans roar and foam. Let the mountains tremble as the waters surge!

Psalm 46:1–3

Chapters 5, 32, 38, 86

"Be still, and know that I am God!"

Psalm 46:10

Chapter 40, 75

Surely God is my help; the Lord is the one who sustains me.

Psalm 54:4 NIV

Chapter 15

Give your burdens to the LORD, and he will take care of you. He will not permit the godly to slip and fall.

Psalm 55:22

Chapter 1

But when I am afraid, I will put my trust in you.

Psalm 56:3

Chapter 28

But as for me, I will sing about your power. Each morning I will sing with joy about your unfailing love. For you have been my refuge, a place of safety when I am in distress.

Psalm 59:16

Chapter 28

O my people, trust in him at all times. Pour out your heart to him, for God is our refuge.

Psalm 62:8

Chapters 77, 83

Your unfailing love is better than life itself; how I praise you! I will praise you as long as I live, lifting up my hands to you in prayer. You satisfy me more than the richest feast. I will praise you with songs of joy. I lie awake thinking of you, meditating on you through the night. Because you are my helper, I sing for joy in the shadow of your wings. I cling to you; your strong right hand holds me securely.

Psalm 63:3–8

Chapters 43, 68 (v. 4)

Then I will praise God's name with singing, and I will honor him with thanksgiving.

Psalm 69:30

Chapters 25, 68

Yet I still belong to you; you hold my right hand. You guide me with your counsel, leading me to a glorious destiny.

Psalm 73:23–24

Chapters 65 (v. 23), 79

This I declare about the LORD: He alone is my refuge, my place of safety; he is my God, and I trust him.

Psalm 91:2

Chapter 54

He will cover you with his feathers, and under his wings you will find refuge.

Psalm 91:4 NIV

Chapter 28

The LORD says, "I will rescue those who love me. I will protect those who trust in my name. When they call on me, I will answer; I will be with them in trouble. I will rescue and honor them. I will reward them with a long life and give them my salvation."

Psalm 91:14–16

Chapter 79

Let all that I am praise the LORD; with my whole heart, I will praise his holy name.

Psalm 103:1

Chapter 68

Search for the LORD and for his strength; continually seek him.

Psalm 105:4

Chapter 88

Everything he does reveals his glory and majesty. His righteousness never fails. He causes us to remember his wonderful works. How gracious and merciful is our LORD!

Psalm 111:3–4

Chapter 47

I have hidden your word in my heart, that I might not sin against you.

Psalm 119:11

Chapter 82

Your word is a lamp to guide my feet and a light for my path.

Psalm 119:105

Chapter 82

I look up to the mountains—does my help come from there? My help comes from the LORD, who made heaven and earth! He will not let you stumble; the one who watches over you will not slumber. Indeed, he who watches over Israel never slumbers or sleeps. The LORD himself watches over you! The LORD stands beside you as your protective shade. The sun will not harm you by day, nor the moon at night. The LORD keeps you from all harm and watches over your life. The LORD keeps watch over you as you come and go, both now and forever.

Psalm 121

Chapters 41, 42 (paraphrased)

Let me hear of your unfailing love each morning, for I am trusting you. Show me where to walk, for I give myself to you.

Psalm 143:8

Chapter 15

The LORD delights in those who fear him, who put their hope in his unfailing love.

Psalm 147:11 NIV

Chapter 3

Trust in the LORD with all your heart; do not depend on your own understanding. Seek his will in all you do, and he will show you which path to take. Don't be impressed with your own wisdom. Instead, fear the LORD and turn away from evil. Then you will have healing for your body and strength for your bones.

Proverbs 3:5–8

Chapters 15 (vv. 5–6), 23 (vv. 5–6), 33, 40 (vv. 5–6), 53 (vv. 5–6)

A glad heart makes a happy face; a broken heart crushes the spirit. A wise person is hungry for knowledge, while the fool feeds on trash. For the despondent, every day brings trouble; for the happy heart, life is a continual feast.

Proverbs 15:13–15

Chapter 83

Pleasant words are like a honeycomb, Sweet and delightful to the soul and healing to the body.

Proverbs 16:24 AMP

Chapter 14

A cheerful heart is good medicine, but a broken spirit saps a person's strength.

Proverbs 17:22

Chapters 21, 83

The LORD directs our steps, so why try to understand everything along the way?

Proverbs 20:24

Chapter 77

For everything there is a season, a time for every activity under heaven. A time to be born and a time to die.

Ecclesiastes 3:1–2

Chapter 57

For everything there is a season, a time for every activity under heaven. . . . A time to cry and a time to laugh. A time to grieve and a time to dance.

Ecclesiastes 3:1, 4

Chapter 84

You will keep in perfect peace all who trust in you, all whose thoughts are fixed on you! Trust in the LORD always, for the LORD GOD is the eternal Rock.

Isaiah 26:3–4

Chapters 6 (v. 3), 12

He gives strength to the weary and increases the power of the weak.

Isaiah 40:29 NIV

Chapter 3

But those who trust in the LORD will find new strength. They will soar high on wings like eagles. They will run and not grow weary. They will walk and not faint.

Isaiah 40:31

Chapter 24

"Don't be afraid, for I am with you. Don't be discouraged, for I am your God. I will strengthen you and help you. I will hold you up with my victorious right hand."

Isaiah 41:10

Chapters 5, 6, 23, 26, 59

"For I hold you by your right hand—I, the LORD your God. And I say to you, 'Don't be afraid. I am here to help you.'"
Isaiah 41:13
Chapters 45, 59

"When you go through deep waters, I will be with you. When you go through rivers of difficulty, you will not drown. When you walk through the fire of oppression, you will not be burned up; the flames will not consume you."
Isaiah 43:2
Chapter 5

"My thoughts are nothing like your thoughts," says the LORD. "And my ways are far beyond anything you could imagine. For just as the heavens are higher than the earth, so my ways are higher than your ways and my thoughts higher than your thoughts."
Isaiah 55:8–9
Chapters 17, 53

The faithful love of the LORD never ends! His mercies never cease. Great is his faithfulness; his mercies begin afresh each morning.
Lamentations 3:22–23
Chapter 36

The LORD is good to those who depend on him, to those who search for him.
Lamentations 3:25
Chapter 73

All around him was a glowing halo, like a rainbow shining in the clouds on a rainy day. This is what the glory of the LORD looked like to me.

Ezekiel 1:28

Chapter 58

If we are thrown into the blazing furnace, the God whom we serve is able to save us. He will rescue us from your power, Your Majesty.

Daniel 3:17

Chapter 44

As for me, I look to the LORD for help. I wait confidently for God to save me, and my God will certainly hear me.

Micah 7:7

Chapter 65

"You are the light of the world—like a city on a hilltop that cannot be hidden. No one lights a lamp and then puts it under a basket. Instead, a lamp is placed on a stand, where it gives light to everyone in the house. In the same way, let your good deeds shine out for all to see, so that everyone will praise your heavenly Father."

Matthew 5:14–16

Chapters 48 (vv. 14–15), 73

"Give us this day our daily bread."

Matthew 6:11 ESV

Chapter 75

"Look at the birds. They don't plant or harvest or store food in barns, for your heavenly Father feeds them. And aren't you far more valuable to him than they are?"

Matthew 6:26

Chapter 24

"And who of you by worrying can add one hour to [the length of] his life?"

Matthew 6:27 AMP

Chapter 49

"So don't worry about tomorrow, for tomorrow will bring its own worries. Today's trouble is enough for today."

Matthew 6:34

Chapters 49, 75

Then Jesus said, "Come to me, all of you who are weary and carry heavy burdens, and I will give you rest."

Matthew 11:28

Chapter 83

Then Peter called to him, "Lord, if it's really you, tell me to come to you, walking on the water." "Yes, come," Jesus said. So Peter went over the side of the boat and walked on the water toward Jesus. But when he saw the strong wind and the waves, he was terrified and began to sink. "Save me, Lord!" he shouted. Jesus immediately reached out and grabbed him. "You have so little faith," Jesus said. "Why did you doubt me?" When they climbed back into the boat, the wind stopped. Then the disciples worshiped him. "You really are the Son of God!" they exclaimed.

Matthew 14:28–33

Chapter 26

Then he said, "I tell you the truth, unless you turn from your sins and become like little children, you will never get into the Kingdom of Heaven."
Matthew 18:3

Chapter 46

Then Jesus went with them to the olive grove called Gethsemane, and he said, "Sit here while I go over there to pray." He took Peter and Zebedee's two sons, James and John, and he became anguished and distressed. He told them, "My soul is crushed with grief to the point of death. Stay here and keep watch with me." He went on a little farther and bowed with his face to the ground, praying, "My Father! If it is possible, let this cup of suffering be taken away from me. Yet I want your will to be done, not mine."
Matthew 26:36–39

Chapters 20 (v. 39), 82

Then Jesus left them a second time and prayed, "My Father! If this cup cannot be taken away unless I drink it, your will be done."
Matthew 26:42

Chapter 82

So he went to pray a third time, saying the same things again.
Matthew 26:44

Chapter 82

"And be sure of this: I am with you always, even to the end of the age."
Matthew 28:20

Chapter 67

"I do believe, but help me overcome my unbelief!"
Mark 9:24
Chapter 77

"And don't be concerned about what to eat and what to drink. Don't worry about such things. . . . Your Father already knows your needs."
Luke 12:29–30
Chapter 24

Now Jesus was telling the disciples a parable to make the point that at all times they ought to pray and not give up and lose heart.
Luke 18:1 AMP
Chapter 19

"For this is how God loved the world: He gave his one and only Son, so that everyone who believes in him will not perish but have eternal life."
John 3:16
Chapter 78

"My sheep listen to my voice."
John 10:27
Chapter 29

"Don't let your hearts be troubled. Trust in God, and trust also in me."
John 14:1
Chapter 83

"I am leaving you with a gift—peace of mind and heart. And the peace I give is a gift the world cannot give. So don't be troubled or afraid."

John 14:27

Chapters 27, 36, 52

"But if you remain in me and my words remain in you, you may ask for anything you want, and it will be granted!"

John 15:7

Chapter 83

"So you have sorrow now, but I will see you again; then you will rejoice, and no one can rob you of that joy."

John 16:22

Chapter 12

"I have told you all this so that you may have peace in me. Here on earth you will have many trials and sorrows. But take heart, because I have overcome the world."

John 16:33

Chapter 81

We can rejoice, too, when we run into problems and trials, for we know that they help us develop endurance. And endurance develops strength of character, and character strengthens our confident hope of salvation. And this hope will not lead to disappointment. For we know how dearly God loves us, because he has given us the Holy Spirit to fill our hearts with his love.

Romans 5:3–5

Chapter 39

But God showed his great love for us by sending Christ to die for us while we were still sinners. And since we have been made right in God's sight by the blood of Christ, he will certainly save us from God's condemnation. For since our friendship with God was restored by the death of his Son while we were still his enemies, we will certainly be saved through the life of his Son. So now we can rejoice in our wonderful new relationship with God because our Lord Jesus Christ has made us friends of God.

Romans 5:8–11

Chapter 66

But if we look forward to something we don't yet have, we must wait patiently and confidently.

Romans 8:25

Epilogue

And we know that God causes everything to work together for the good of those who love God and are called according to his purpose for them.

Romans 8:28

Chapters 20, 39, 60

And we know [with great confidence] that God [who is deeply concerned about us] causes all things to work together [as a plan] for good for those who love God, to those who are called according to His plan and purpose.

Romans 8:28 AMP

Chapter 85

Can anything ever separate us from Christ's love? Does it mean he no longer loves us if we have trouble or calamity, or are persecuted, or hungry, or destitute, or in danger, or threatened with death? (As the Scriptures say, "For your sake we are killed every day; we are being slaughtered like sheep.") No, despite all these things, overwhelming victory is ours through Christ, who loved us. And I am convinced that nothing can ever separate us from God's love. Neither death nor life, neither angels nor demons, neither our fears for today nor our worries about tomorrow—not even the powers of hell can separate us from God's love. No power in the sky above or in the earth below—indeed, nothing in all creation will ever be able to separate us from the love of God that is revealed in Christ Jesus our Lord.

Romans 8:35–39

Chapters 5 (vv. 37–39), 46, 87

If you openly declare that Jesus is Lord and believe in your heart that God raised him from the dead, you will be saved. For it is by believing in your heart that you are made right with God, and it is by openly declaring your faith that you are saved.

Romans 10:9–10

Chapter 61

So we, who are many, are [nevertheless just] one body in Christ, and individually [we are] parts one of another [mutually dependent on each other].

Romans 12:5 AMP

Chapter 9

Never lagging behind in diligence; aglow in the Spirit, enthusiastically serving the Lord; constantly rejoicing in hope [because of our confidence in Christ], steadfast and patient in distress, devoted to prayer [continually seeking wisdom, guidance, and strength].

Romans 12:11–12 AMP

Chapters 52, 64

Rejoice in hope, be patient in tribulation, be constant in prayer.

Romans 12:12 ESV

Chapter 4

I pray that God, the source of hope, will fill you completely with joy and peace because you trust in him. Then you will overflow with confident hope through the power of the Holy Spirit.

Romans 15:13

Chapters 38, 72

May the God of hope fill you with all joy and peace in believing, so that by the power of the Holy Spirit you may abound in hope.

Romans 15:13 ESV

Chapter 71

May the God of hope fill you with all joy and peace in believing [through the experience of your faith] that by the power of the Holy Spirit you will abound in hope and overflow with confidence in His promises.

Romans 15:13 AMP

Chapters 45 (paraphrased), 47

No temptation has overtaken you that is not common to man. God is faithful, and he will not let you be tempted beyond your ability, but with the temptation he will also provide the way of escape, that you may be able to endure it.

1 Corinthians 10:13 ESV

Chapter 69

Be on guard. Stand firm in the faith. Be courageous. Be strong.

1 Corinthians 16:13

Chapter 34

All praise to God, the Father of our Lord Jesus Christ. God is our merciful Father and the source of all comfort. He comforts us in all our troubles so that we can comfort others. When they are troubled, we will be able to give them the same comfort God has given us.

2 Corinthians 1:3–4

Chapters 21, 60, 63, Epilogue

Therefore we do not lose heart. Though outwardly we are wasting away, yet inwardly we are being renewed day by day. For our light and momentary troubles are achieving for us an eternal glory that far outweighs them all. So we fix our eyes not on what is seen, but on what is unseen, since what is seen is temporary, but what is unseen is eternal.

2 Corinthians 4:16–18 NIV

Chapter 51

For we walk by faith, not by sight [living our lives in a manner consistent with our confident belief in God's promises].

2 Corinthians 5:7 AMP

Chapter 38

Each time he said, "My grace is all you need. My power works best in weakness." So now I am glad to boast about my weaknesses, so that the power of Christ can work through me.

2 Corinthians 12:9

Chapter 74

Share each other's burdens, and in this way obey the law of Christ.

Galatians 6:2

Chapters 8, 70

Carry one another's burdens and in this way you will fulfill the requirements of the law of Christ [that is, the law of Christian love].

Galatians 6:2 AMP

Chapters 9, 63

Therefore, whenever we have the opportunity, we should do good to everyone—especially to those in the family of faith.

Galatians 6:10

Chapter 70

All praise to God, the Father of our Lord Jesus Christ, who has blessed us with every spiritual blessing in the heavenly realms because we are united with Christ.

Ephesians 1:3

Chapter 68

Be kind to each other, tenderhearted, forgiving one another, just as God through Christ has forgiven you.

Ephesians 4:32

Chapter 50

Be strong in the Lord [draw your strength from Him and be empowered through your union with Him] and in the power of His [boundless] might.

Ephesians 6:10 AMP

Chapter 18

Put on all of God's armor so that you will be able to stand firm against all strategies of the devil.

Ephesians 6:11

Chapter 56

Therefore, put on every piece of God's armor so you will be able to resist the enemy in the time of evil. Then after the battle you will still be standing firm. Stand your ground, putting on the belt of truth and the body armor of God's righteousness. For shoes, put on the peace that comes from the Good News so that you will be fully prepared. In addition to all of these, hold up the shield of faith to stop the fiery arrows of the devil. Put on salvation as your helmet, and take the sword of the Spirit, which is the word of God.

Ephesians 6:13–17

Chapter 21

Pray in the Spirit at all times and on every occasion. Stay alert and be persistent in your prayers for all believers everywhere.

Ephesians 6:18

Chapter 8

He who began a good work in you will carry it on to completion.

Philippians 1:6 NIV

Chapter 27

It is my own eager expectation and hope, that [looking toward the future] I will not disgrace myself nor be ashamed in anything, but that with courage and the utmost freedom of speech, even now as always, Christ will be magnified and exalted in my body, whether by life or by death.

Philippians 1:20 AMP

Chapter 64

Don't look out only for your own interests, but take an interest in others, too.

Philippians 2:4

Chapter 70

For it is [not your strength, but it is] God who is effectively at work in you, both to will and to work [that is, strengthening, energizing, and creating in you the longing and the ability to fulfill your purpose] for His good pleasure.

Philippians 2:13 AMP

Chapter 44

I press on to reach the end of the race and receive the heavenly prize for which God, through Christ Jesus, is calling us.

Philippians 3:14

Chapter 75

Always be full of joy in the Lord. I say it again—rejoice! Let everyone see that you are considerate in all you do. Remember, the Lord is coming soon. Don't worry about anything; instead, pray about everything. Tell God what you need, and thank him for all he has done. Then you will experience God's peace, which exceeds anything we can understand. His peace will guard your hearts and minds as you live in Christ Jesus.

Philippians 4:4–7

Chapters 7, 16 (v. 6), 17 (v. 6 paraphrased), 44 (v. 6), 69 (vv. 6–7)

Do not be anxious or worried about anything, but in everything [every circumstance and situation] by prayer and petition with thanksgiving, continue to make your [specific] requests known to God. And the peace of God [that peace which reassures the heart, that peace] which transcends all understanding, [that peace which] stands guard over your hearts and your minds in Christ Jesus [is yours].

Philippians 4:6–7 AMP

Chapter 55

Don't worry about anything; instead, pray about everything. Tell God what you need, and thank him for all he has done. Then you will experience God's peace, which exceeds anything we can understand. His peace will guard your hearts and minds as you live in Christ Jesus. And now, dear brothers and sisters, one final thing. Fix your thoughts on what is true, and honorable, and right, and pure, and lovely, and admirable. Think about things that are excellent and worthy of praise. Keep putting into practice all you learned and received from me—everything you heard from me and saw me doing. Then the God of peace will be with you.

Philippians 4:6–9

Chapters 10 (v. 8), 22, 31 (v. 8), 62 (vv.8 –9)

I have learned how to be content with whatever I have.

Philippians 4:11

Chapter 72

I can do all things [which He has called me to do] through Him who strengthens and empowers me [to fulfill His purpose—I am self-sufficient in Christ's sufficiency; I am ready for anything and equal to anything through Him who infuses me with inner strength and confident peace].

Philippians 4:13 AMP

Chapter 4

We also pray that you will be strengthened with all his glorious power so you will have all the endurance and patience you need. May you be filled with joy, always thanking the Father. He has enabled you to share in the inheritance that belongs to his people, who live in the light.

Colossians 1:11–12

Chapters 21, 72

You were dead because of your sins and because your sinful nature was not yet cut away. Then God made you alive with Christ, for he forgave all our sins. He canceled the record of the charges against us and took it away by nailing it to the cross.

Colossians 2:13–14

Chapter 78

Conduct yourself with wisdom in your interactions with outsiders (non-believers), make the most of each opportunity [treating it as something precious].

Colossians 4:5 AMP

Chapter 74

So encourage each other and build each other up.

1 Thessalonians 5:11

Chapter 16

Be unceasing and persistent in prayer.

1 Thessalonians 5:17 AMP

Chapter 19

Be thankful in all circumstances, for this is God's will for you who belong to Christ Jesus.

1 Thessalonians 5:18

Chapter 68

In every situation [no matter what the circumstances] be thankful and continually give thanks to God; for this is the will of God for you in Christ Jesus.

1 Thessalonians 5:18 AMP

Chapter 10

I urge you, first of all, to pray for all people. Ask God to help them; intercede on their behalf, and give thanks for them.

1 Timothy 2:1

Chapters 8, 63

For God has not given us a spirit of fear and timidity, but of power, love, and self-discipline.

2 Timothy 1:7

Chapter 69

This hope is a strong and trustworthy anchor for our souls. It leads us through the curtain into God's inner sanctuary. Jesus has already gone in there for us.

Hebrews 6:19–20

Chapter 57

Let us hold fast the confession of our hope without wavering, for he who promised is faithful.

Hebrews 10:23 ESV

Chapter 66

Let us seize and hold tightly the confession of our hope without wavering, for He who promised is reliable and trustworthy and faithful [to His word].

Hebrews 10:23 AMP

Chapter 84

Now faith is the assurance (title deed, confirmation) of things hoped for (divinely guaranteed), and the evidence of things not seen [the conviction of their reality—faith comprehends as fact what cannot be experienced by the physical senses].

Hebrews 11:1 AMP

Chapter 58

And let us run with endurance the race God has set before us. We do this by keeping our eyes on Jesus, the champion who initiates and perfects our faith. Because of the joy awaiting him, he endured the cross, disregarding its shame. Now he is seated in the place of honor beside God's throne.

Hebrews 12:1–2

Chapters 20 (v. 2), 25

For God has said, "I will never fail you. I will never abandon you."

Hebrews 13:5

Chapter 30

Whatever is good and perfect is a gift coming down to us from God our Father, who created all the lights in the heavens.

James 1:17

Chapters 43, 68

So humble yourselves before God. Resist the devil, and he will flee from you. Come close to God, and God will come close to you.

James 4:7–8

Chapters 7, 55 (v. 7)

Submit yourselves, then, to God. Resist the devil, and he will flee from you. Come near to God and he will come near to you.

James 4:7–8 NIV

Chapter 81

Is anyone among you sick? Let them call the elders of the church to pray over them and anoint them with oil in the name of the Lord.

James 5:14 NIV

Chapter 10

Confess your sins to each other and pray for each other so that you may be healed. The earnest prayer of a righteous person has great power and produces wonderful results.

James 5:16

Chapters 8, 41

Therefore, confess your sins to one another [your false steps, your offenses], and pray for one another, that you may be healed and restored. The heartfelt and persistent prayer of a righteous man (believer) can accomplish much [when put into action and made effective by God—it is dynamic and can have tremendous power].

James 5:16 AMP

Chapter 19

Through Christ you have come to trust in God. And you have placed your faith and hope in God because he raised Christ from the dead and gave him great glory.

1 Peter 1:21

Chapter 76

Your adornment must not be merely external—with interweaving and elaborate knotting of the hair, and wearing gold jewelry, or [being superficially preoccupied with] dressing in expensive clothes; but let it be [the inner beauty of] the hidden person of the heart, with the imperishable quality and unfading charm of a gentle and peaceful spirit, [one that is calm and self-controlled, not overanxious, but serene and spiritually mature] which is very precious in the sight of God.

1 Peter 3:3–4 AMP

Chapter 80

"The eyes of the Lord watch over those who do right, and his ears are open to their prayers."

1 Peter 3:12

Chapter 75

Casting all your cares [all your anxieties, all your worries, and all your concerns, once and for all] on Him, for He cares about you [with deepest affection, and watches over you very carefully].

1 Peter 5:7 AMP

Chapters 13, 37

Stay alert! Watch out for your great enemy, the devil. He prowls around like a roaring lion, looking for someone to devour. Stand firm against him, and be strong in your faith.

1 Peter 5:8–9

Chapters 1, 7, 55 (v. 8)

After you have suffered a little while, he will restore, support, and strengthen you, and he will place you on a firm foundation.

1 Peter 5:10

Chapter 72

The one who is in you [Jesus] is greater than the one who is in the world [Satan].

1 John 4:4 NIV

Chapter 26

Little children, you are from God and have overcome them, for he who is in you is greater than he who is in the world.

1 John 4:4 ESV

Chapter 77

We know how much God loves us, and we have put our trust in his love. God is love, and all who live in love live in God, and God lives in them.

1 John 4:16

Chapter 15

I have no greater joy than to hear that my children are walking in the truth.

3 John 1:4 NIV

Chapter 3

And instantly I was in the Spirit, and I saw a throne in heaven and someone sitting on it. The one sitting on the throne was as brilliant as gemstones—like jasper and carnelian. And the glow of an emerald circled his throne like a rainbow.

Revelation 4:2–3

Chapter 58